50 LANDMARK PAPERS

every

Pediatric Surgeon Should Know

This book identifies the 50 key scientific articles in the field of pediatric surgery. It provides a commentary to each carefully selected paper and explains why these papers are so important, thus providing every surgeon with the foundation stones of knowledge in this fast-moving area.

The key advances in neonatal, pediatric and fetal surgery – game-changers if you will – that have led to the significant improvements in clinical outcome and results are all included. The choice of papers provides an insight into the development of pediatric surgery and offers an important aid to understanding the subject for practicing pediatric surgeons and residents.

50 Landmark Papers Series

50 Landmark Papers Every Spine Surgeon Should Know
Alexander R Vaccaro, Charles G Fisher and Jefferson R Wilson

50 Landmark Papers Every Trauma Surgeon Should Know
Stephen M Cohn and Ara J Feinstein

50 Landmark Papers Every Acute Care Surgeon Should Know
Stephen M Cohn and Peter Rhee

50 Landmark Papers Every Vascular and Endovascular Surgeon Should Know
Juan Carlos Jimenez and Samuel Eric Wilson

50 Landmark Papers Every Oral and Maxillofacial Surgeon Should Know
Niall MH McLeod and Peter A Brennan

50 Landmark Papers Every Intensivist Should Know
Stephen M Cohn, Alan Lisbon and Stephen Heard

50 Landmark Papers Every Thyroid and Parathyroid Surgeon Should Know
Sam Wiseman and Sebastian Aspinall

50 Landmark Papers Every Pediatric Surgeon Should Know
Mark Davenport, Bashar Aldeiri and Joseph Davidson

For more information about this series, please visit www.routledge.com/
50-Landmark-Papers/book-series/50LP

50 LANDMARK PAPERS

every
Pediatric Surgeon Should Know

EDITED BY

Mark Davenport ChM FRCS (Paeds) FRCS (Eng) FRCPS (Glas)

Consultant Paediatric Surgeon and Professor of Paediatric Surgery
Department of Paediatric Surgery, Kings College Hospital, London

Bashar Aldeiri MD PhD FRCS (Paeds)

Consultant Paediatric Surgeon
Department of Paediatric Surgery, Chelsea and Westminster Hospital, London

Joseph Davidson MA MBBS MRCS

Specialist Registrar and Research Fellow
Department of Paediatric Surgery, Great Ormond Street Hospital, London

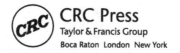

CRC Press
Taylor & Francis Group
Boca Raton London New York

CRC Press is an imprint of the
Taylor & Francis Group, an **informa** business

First edition published 2024
by CRC Press
6000 Broken Sound Parkway NW, Suite 300, Boca Raton, FL 33487-2742

and by CRC Press
4 Park Square, Milton Park, Abingdon, Oxon, OX14 4RN

CRC Press is an imprint of Taylor & Francis Group, LLC

ISBN: 9781032377872 (hbk)
ISBN: 9781032371221 (pbk)
ISBN: 9781003341901 (ebk)

DOI: 10.1201/9781003341901

Typeset in Times
by KnowledgeWorks Global Ltd.

Contents

Editor Biographies

Prof. Mark Davenport ChM FRCS (Eng) FRCPS (Glas) FRCS (Paeds)

Mark Davenport qualified in medicine in 1981 from the University of Leeds with surgical training at Leeds, Sheffield, Manchester and London, before arriving finally as a consultant in 1994 at King's College Hospital, London, in 1994. There, he completed a postgraduate research degree (ChM) and since 2008 became a professor of pediatric surgery at King's College, London.

His main clinical interests are hepatobiliary diseases such as biliary atresia and choledochal malformation together with the surgery of the short gut.

He has been an editor for the *Journal of Pediatric Surgery* since 2008 and has written two editions of two general pediatric surgery textbooks, an international multiauthor specialist book on pediatric liver and pancreatic disease and the eighth edition of the popular Rob & Smith's *Operative Pediatric Surgery*.

He was elected president of the British Association of Paediatric Surgeons (BAPS) for 2016–2018.

Mr. Bashar Aldeiri MD PhD FRCS (Eng)

Bashar Aldeiri is a consultant pediatric and neonatal surgeon at Chelsea and Westminster and Imperial College London. Bashar qualified from Damascus University School of Medicine, Syria, in 2006, and attained pediatric surgical training in Damascus, Manchester, London and Southampton. In 2014, he secured the Constance Thornley research fellowship at the University of Manchester, where he achieved a doctorate in philosophy in 2018. In his thesis, he looked at the development of the ventral body wall in mammals and distinct developmental pathways that lead to failure of body wall closure and the development of an exomphalos anomaly.

His main areas of clinical interests are pediatric upper gastrointestinal surgery and neonatal surgery.

Mr. Joseph Davidson MA MBBS MRCS

Joe Davidson completed his medical degree from New College, Oxford and King's College London Medical School, qualifying in 2014. In 2016, he commenced an academic training program in pediatric surgery and has trained at King's College

Hospital, Evelina London Children's Hospital and Great Ormond Street Hospital, where he is currently completing a PhD in fetal immunology at the University College London Great Ormond Street Institute of Child Health (UCL-GOS ICH).

He has research interests in long-term outcomes in surgical patients as well as a passion for integrating cutting-edge basic science techniques to improve understanding of surgical pathology and treatment.

Preface

This is a subject which will inevitably stimulate controversy and argument. How do you choose a Landmark?

We set out to include published papers that impact on the practice of our specialty. There must be, of course, some historical contributions which have entered the fabric of our surgery – so choosing Conrad von Rammstedt, Cameron Haight and Orvar Swenson's contributions (Chapters 1–3) were no-brainers. Some clearly wrote their own recommendation with innovative approaches to surgical anatomy that certainly changed practice. Puri and O'Donnell's STING procedure (Chapter 38) altering the vesicoureteric junction; Peña's (and DeVries') novel approach to the anorectum (Chapter 23); and Adrian Bianchi's original interpretation of the arterial arcades of the jejunum (Chapter 15). We then tried to think in terms of our various family members: urology; neonatal; oncology, etc. Which ones changed or became the keystone of today's practice – such as the work of Paul Mitrofanof (Chapter 40) and Padraig Malone (Chapter 39) in urology and Bell et al.'s classification for neonatal necrotizing enterocolitis (NEC) (Chapter 17) and Helen Noblett's rectal biopsy suction apparatus (Chapter 20) in gastrointestinal surgery are great examples of this. Others perhaps are a bit more esoteric, such as Judah Folkman and tumour biology (Chapter 48) or Stanley Dudrick and the genesis of parenteral nutrition (Chapter 44).

Where we differ markedly from other books in this Surgical Landmarks series is in the lack of truly scientific evidence for much of our practice! In the late twentieth century, the randomized controlled clinical trial became the preferred instrument and arbiter of surgical practice, certainly in oncology surgery and the like but not so much in pediatric surgery. Why? Well, we have by comparison so few patients to put into trials, and even then there is a great resistance from the surgical community, who lack equipoise or parents who run shy of recruitment. The Landmark randomized trials in this book are few (e.g., the MOMS trial, the TOTAL trial and the PLUTO trial are great examples in fetal intervention studies, as discussed in Chapters 5–7), but there are also a pyloric stenosis trial (Chapter 10) and an NEC trial (Chapter 18). Notably, all had difficulty recruiting, and for some their results are still arguable and less clear-cut than had been hoped for.

We undoubtedly have an Anglo-centric, trans-Atlantic bias, but in medicine dating from the late twentieth century this is overwhelmingly true of most reviews. There are only three foreign language contributions (Rammstedt, Kasai and Mitrofanoff, in Chapters 1, 25 and 40), and with abject apologies, none from Latin America, Russia or China.

Currently, the most cited paper in the pediatric surgical literature appears to be the 1996 paper in the *Journal of Pediatric Surgery* by Metkus et al. (Chapter 4), "Sonographic Predictors of Survival in Fetal Diaphragmatic Hernia," which used ultrasound to prenatally diagnose congenital diaphragmatic hernia (CDH) and characterise and correlate several anatomical features with outcome and survival of infants culminating in the lung-to-head ratio. This we reasoned was indeed a Landmark in providing objective and prognosis information in an area where so much had been subjective and magical, and it pointed the way ultimately to the TOTAL trial. The second most cited paper has been a single-author review by Lewis Spitz (1) in 2007, presenting detailed etiology, pathophysiology, diagnosis, treatment, outcomes and complications of esophageal atresia. This manuscript is obviously a Level V evidence review, but popular though such reviews are, it really falls outside of our criteria for inclusion here.

Sullivan et al. (2) took a different route to try to identify "disruptive" papers. This involved not simply counting the number of citations, but designing a more complex formula bringing in what was written before and then after in the field. Papers such as Gauderer's PEG device (Chapter 13) and the Bell NEC classification (Chapter 17) still enter the Top Ten here, but the criteria also result in some strange entries on 'Bicycle Injuries in Calgary' (4) and 'Internet Use in *children requiring cardiac surgery* ...' (5). Such papers are probably no ones' (even the authors', dare I say it) idea of Landmarks!

In conclusion, if this does not spark conversation and debate, then we have not done our jobs properly. We hope at least readers will find the ones they know about but also the golden nuggets of the ones that got away.

The Editors

REFERENCES

1. Spitz L. Oesophageal atresia. Orphanet J Rare Dis. 2007;2:24.
2. Sullivan G, Skertich NJ, Gulack BC, Becerraa AZ, Shahb AN. Shifting paradigms: The top 100 most disruptive papers in core pediatric surgery journals. J Pediatr Surg. 2021;56:1263–127.
3. Guichon DM, Myles ST. Bicycle injuries: One-year sample in Calgary. J Trauma. 1975;15:504–6.
4. Ikemba CM, Kozinetz CA, Feltes TF, Fraser CD Jr, et al. Internet use in families with children requiring cardiac surgery for congenital heart disease. Pediatrics. 2002;109(3):419–22.

Contributors

Adrian Bianchi
St Mary's Hospital
Manchester, UK

Michael WL Gauderer
Salem, South Carolina, USA

George W Holcomb III

Padraig Malone

Sean Marven
Sheffield Children's Hospital
Sheffield, UK

Masaki Nio
Tohoku University Graduate School of
   Medicine
Seiryo-machi, Aoba-ku, Japan

Mikko P Pakarinen
Pediatric Liver and Gut Research Group
Children's Hospital
University of Helsinki and Helsinki
   University Hospital
Helsinki, Finland

Prem Puri
University College Dublin
Dublin, Ireland

Risto Rintala
Children's Hospital
University of Helsinki and Helsinki
   University Hospital
Helsinki, Finland

Steven S Rothenberg
Paediatric Surgeon and Minimally
   Invasive Surgery Center
Rocky Mountain Childrens Hospital
Denver, Colorado, USA

Naomi Wright
King's Centre for Global Health
   and Health Partnerships
London, UK

Atsuyuki Yamataka
Department of Pediatric Surgery
Juntendo University School of Medicine
Tokyo, Japan

CHAPTER 1

Zur Operation der angeborenen Pylorusstenose

Conrad von Rammstedt

Medizinische Klinik 1912:1702–1706.

BACKGROUND AND ABSTRACT

Hypertrophic pyloric stenosis in infants was only relatively recently described with
a famous presentation of two cases by Harald Hirschsprung in 1888 in Copenhagen
identifying the key clinical features of projectile vomiting in the first few weeks
of life and a palpable pyloric tumour. Following this, a whole variety of surgical
manoeuvres were suggested, but cynical physicians often preferred to persist with
medical remedies such as belladonna (atropine), cocaine and opium while maintaining
nutrition with things like milk and saline enemas.

The paper itself starts by critiquing the physicians' approach, urging them to refer 'in
timely fashion, or at least before they lapse into an unfortunate wretched condition'.
Rammstedt then goes on to reject direct operations on the pylorus such as pyloric
resection, not-internal splitting of the stenosis by an instrument inserted via a
gastrostomy and the Heineke–Mikulicz pyloroplasty. He doesn't have much time
for gastrojejunostomy, then in vogue across the
Atlantic. He identifies the crucial problem in small,
sick infants – that of leakage with peritonitis almost
certainly resulting in death (Figure 1.1).

His solution builds upon the work of Wilhelm Weber
(1) and later Dufour and Fredet, who had done partial
pyloroplasties but left the mucosa intact. Rammstedt's
contribution was to leave the mucosa intact.

So, on August 23, 1911, at the Rafael Clinic in Munster,
Germany, Rammstedt operated on a seven-week-
old infant. 'After cutting through the hypertrophied,
bloodless muscle, it occurred to me that the stenosis
was relieved'. He then actually goes on to try and
replicate the Weber partial pyloroplasty, but the sutures
kept cutting out, so he left it open, mucosa gaping. The
child had a fairly stormy postoperative course with
recurrent vomiting but was discharged by day 8.

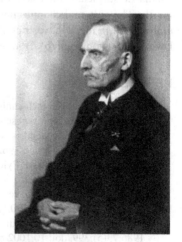

Figure 1.1 Conrad Von
Rammstedt. (Courtesy of the
National Library of Medicine.)

DOI: 10.1201/9781003341901-1

His second case was operated upon almost a year later in 1912 and didn't include any attempt at pyloric reconstruction. There was no postoperative problems and set the scene for this operation to become the definitive one for pyloric stenosis.

It is noteworthy that the paper spells the author's name with an extra *m*. This was the way he spelt his name at the time but later changed in favour of the shorter version when he discovered an error in transcribing family records. This is the version of the name that tends to be used nowadays – Ramstedt. It is also interesting to note that back at the time of his first operation, he never had never seen a case of pyloric stenosis and was probably pushed into it as the child was the firstborn of a noble family from the vicinity. Ram(m) stedt had a long, eventful career, being a military surgeon on the Western Front in the Great War and operating well into his 70s, before finally dying at the age of 96 in 1963.

IMPACT (MARK DAVENPORT)

Pyloromyotomy for pyloric stenosis fairly quickly became the standard operation, though was not without its critics. For instance, Mr Robert Ramsay became the first person to perform it in the UK, at the Belgrave Hospital in Lambeth, London, in July 1918. Unfortunately, the child died one week later, though the stenosis was shown to have been relieved at postmortem. Still, he persevered, although five out of his first ten infants died. He attributed this to poor nutrition and dehydration rather than the operation and went on to have a personal series of over 200. Even so, there were pockets of resistance, and Jacoby was able to report 195 cases managed up until 1960, in which medical treatment was favoured based on atropine methylnitrate (Eumydrin™) with a success rate of about 50% (2).

Today, over 100 years since that first operation (3, 4) it is still the operation that paediatric surgical trainees cut their teeth on and can count themselves as part of our family. The only real changes have been in surgical access. In the 1980s, a circum-umbilical skin incision was popularised (5), and in the 2000s we had the advent of a laparoscopic approach (6). Both give excellent cosmetic access.

REFERENCES

1. Weber W. Ueber einem Technische Neuerung bei der Operation der Pylorus des Sauglings. Berlin Klin Wchschr. 1910;47:763.
2. Jacoby NM. Pyloric stenosis: selective medical and surgical treatment. A survey of sixteen years' experience. Lancet. 1962;1:119–21.
3. Georgoula C, Gardiner M. Pyloric stenosis a 100 years after Ramstedt. Arch Dis Child. 2012;97:741–45.
4. Shaw A. Ramstedt and the centennial of pyloromyotomy. J Pediatr Surg. 2012;47(7):1433–35. doi: 10.1016/j.jpedsurg.2012.06.002. PMID: 22813809.
5. Tan KC, Bianchi A. Circumumbilical incision for pyloromyotomy. Br J Surg. 1986;73(5):399. doi: 10.1002/bjs.1800730529. PMID: 3708297.
6. Hall NJ, Pacilli M, Eaton S, Reblock K, Gaines BA, et al. Recovery after open versus laparoscopic pyloromyotomy for pyloric stenosis: a double-blind multicentre randomised controlled trial. Lancet. 2009;373(9661):390–98. doi: 10.1016/S0140-6736(09)60006-4

Congenital Atresia of the Esophagus with Tracheoesophageal Fistula: Extrapleural Ligation of Fistula and End-to-End Anastomosis of Esophageal Segments

Cameron Haight and Harry Towsley

Surgery Gynecology and Obstetrics 1943; 76:672–688.

BACKGROUND AND ABSTRACT

This epoch-making event happened in Ann Arbor, Michigan, in March 1941 and followed a series of failures of attempted primary repairs of esophageal atresias (EA). The only survivors previously had been staged repairs using skin-lined tubes created subcutaneously joining cervical esophagostomies to the stomach.

The patient, a baby girl, had been driven over 600 miles from the upper reaches of the state and was 12 days old with a documented birth weight of 8 lbs 4 ozs (3.66 kg). The initial X-rays show a grossly distended stomach and even some contrast below the diaphragm as overspill via the fistula from some instilled into the upper pouch. Anaesthesia was initially just local for the thoracotomy and then ether for the anastomosis. An antibiotic (sulfathiazole) was given by rectum. There were some unusual elements of the operation in that Haight (Figure 2.1) approached the EA and fistula via a left-sided extrapleural thoracotomy involving rib resections. The anastomosis was performed using 'fine silk'. In later years, he developed an unusual telescoping two-layer anastomotic technique.

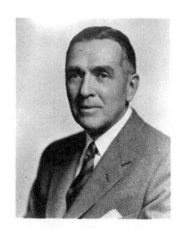

Of course, there was a leak, but it was contained as it was extrapleural and was short-lived with resolution by the 20th day. A gastrostomy had been added that provided the nutritional input until oral feeds were started. The patient also developed a stricture requiring a dilatation at 17 months and spent over 20 months in hospital before final discharge home.

Figure 2.1 Cameron Haight, ca. 1958; HS10730. (Courtesy of University of Michigan Library Digital Collections. Accessed February 11, 2023.)

DOI: 10.1201/9781003341901-2

We even have long-term follow-up information about the patient as Dr Haight included details of her at the age of 16 years in a Presidential Address to the American Association for Thoracic Surgery, where he also described his personal series of over 200 cases to the audience (1). A few years further on, in 2005, the patient was referenced again, now well over 60 and having had her own son.

REFERENCE

1. Haight C. Some observations on esophageal atresias and tracheo-esophageal fistulas of congenital origin. J Thoracic Surg. 1957;34:141–172.

CHAPTER 3

Resection of Rectum and Rectosigmoid with Preservation of the Sphincter for Benign Spastic Lesions Producing Megacolon. An Experimental Study

Orvar Swenson and Alexander H. Bill Jr.

Surgery 1948; 24: 212–220.

ABSTRACT

1. A series of 20 cases of megacolon with spasm of the rectosigmoid in children is reported.
2. A method of resection of the rectum and rectosigmoid, with preservation of the sphincter, is described. This method was evaluated in a series of 15 dogs. Results showed (a) infection in but one case, (b) good sphincter control in all and (c) no postoperative strictures.
3. The operation has been successfully used on three children.

COMMENTARY (MARK DAVENPORT)

It is helpful that we have Swenson's own commentary on his Landmark work (1) to aid appreciation of this work.

Previous attempts at a curative operation for a condition described 60 years previously by Harald Hirschsprung ('Sluggishness of the Stool in the Newborn, Resulting from Dilatation and Hypertrophy of the Colon') (2) had floundered on an imperfect understanding of what exactly was going on. Sir Frederick Treves had got nearest with a resection of all the distal bowel and anal sphincter bringing the proximal bowel out effectively as a perineal stoma (3).

Ovar Swenson (Figure 3.1) was on staff at Boston Children's Hospital and had been treating many children with Hirschsprung's disease as well as performing colonic manometric studies on a number. He describes one key case, a six-year-old boy where

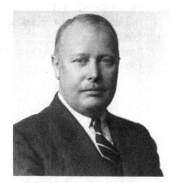

Figure 3.1 Orvar Swenson (1909–2012). (Courtesy of the National Library of Medicine.)

DOI: 10.1201/9781003341901-3

he used a diverting colostomy, which 'cured' the child and was unable to show any sign of peristalsis in the distal limb. Barium studies invariably showed distal segmental contractions right down to the anus. Convinced that the distal colon was the source of the problem he perfected the technique of resection and low colo-anal anastomosis in a series of dogs before undertaking this on June 19, 1947, with closure of the colostomy two months later. Dr Swenson later reported that this index patient was 'now a 48-year-old married man with four children!' Two further cases were reported with equally gratifying results.

That period was epochal in terms of Hirschsprung's disease in that both the reports of Zuelzer and Wilson (Detroit and Michigan respectively) (4), and Whitehouse and Kernohan (Rochester, Minnesota) (5) were published in that same year, showing an absence of ganglion cells in the distal rectosigmoid and thus providing a histological basis for Swenson's work.

Today, this operation is relatively infrequently performed by surgeons because of worries of nerve, seminal vesicle and vasal injury inherent in a low pelvic dissection in the male. Using the same Swenson principle, first Bernard Duhamel (6) and then the various modifications of the operation pioneered by Franco Soave (7) emerged as more popular options.

REFERENCES

1. Swenson O. My early experience with Hirschsprung's disease. J Pediatr Surg. 1989;24:839–845.
2. Hirschsprung H. Stuhlträgheit Neugeborener in Folge von Dilatation und Hypertrophie des Colons. Jahrb f Kinderh. 1886;27:1–7.
3. Treves F. Idiopathic dilatation of the colon. Lancet. 1898;(i):276–279.
4. Zuelzer WW, Wilson JL. Functional intestinal obstruction on a congenital neurogenic basis in infancy. Am J Dis Child. 1948;75:40–64.
5. Whitehouse ER, Kernohan JW. Myenteric plexus in congenital megacolon. Arch Intern Med. 1948;82:75–111.
6. Duhamel B. A new operation for the treatment of Hirschsprung's disease. Arch Dis Child. 1960;35:38–39.
7. Soave F. Hirschsprung's disease. A new surgical technique. Arch Dis Child. 1964;39:116–124.

CHAPTER 4

Sonographic Predictors of Survival in Fetal Diaphragmatic Hernia

Andrea P Metkus, Roy A Filly, Mark D Stringer,
Michael R Harrison, and N Scott Adzick

Journal of Pediatric Surgery 1996; 31: 148–151.
Citations $n = 577$

ABSTRACT

The authors studied the predictive value of detailed fetal sonographic parameters
on outcomes for 55 patients with prenatally diagnosed congenital diaphragmatic
hernia managed at an extracorporeal membrane oxygenation (ECMO) center. Their
sonographic assessment included gestational age at time of diagnosis, polyhydramnios
(largest amniotic fluid pocket diameter), presence of liver and/or stomach herniation
and abdominal circumference at the level of the umbilical cord. They measured the
right-lung two-dimensional area at the level of the atria as an estimate of lung size
and mediastinal shift. The ratio of right lung area to head circumference (LHR) was
calculated to minimize lung size differences owing to gestational age. The principal
outcome variable was survival. The overall survival rate was 65%. If the diagnosis
was made after 25 weeks' gestation, the survival rate was 100% (12 of 12); the
rate was 56% if the diagnosis was made at or before 25 weeks (P < 0.005). All five
neonates with an LHR of < 0.6 died; the survival rate was 100% for those whose
LHR was > 1.35; and those with an LHR between 0.6 and 1.35 had a 61% survival
rate (P < 0.001). The survival rate for those whose liver was not herniated was 100%
(10 of 10); herniation of the liver decreased the survival rate to 56% (P < 0.05).

Stomach position, polyhydramnios and abdominal circumference were not found
to be useful survival predictors. No prenatal sonographic parameter was absolutely
predictive of postnatal death except very small right lung size, which was present in
only five of the 55 patients. Survival is highly likely if the liver is not herniated into
the thorax and/or the right lung is large.

COMMENTARY (MARK DAVENPORT)

This series is from the original Fetal Treatment Center in San Francisco led by
Michael Harrison, though Roy Filly clearly deserves much credit as the actual
ultrasonologist doing the scans. They sought to establish a practical prognostic score
for evaluation of the antenatally detected congenital diaphragmatic hernia (CDH). The
area of the good (i.e., right) lung at a particular ultrasound plane ('four-chamber view')

DOI: 10.1201/9781003341901-4

was evaluated and corrected for gestational age using the head circumference, leading to the simple ratio (lung to head ratio – LHR) where low was poor and high was good. They also used this paper to reinforce the poor prognostic feature of herniation of the liver into the left thoracic space. It is also important to recognize that this study was a highly selected sample from a much larger referral cohort to San Francisco ($n = 176$) – the key to inclusion being the isolated nature of the CDH.

The LHR quickly became the way to evaluate the fetal diaphragmatic hernia, and its use rapidly spread to other fetal medicine units throughout the world.

LHR was used as the arbiter of the subsequent San Francisco Fetoscopic Endoluminal Tracheal Occlusion (FETO) trial (1) but was found wanting there when accurate discrimination of the fetuses with a truly poor prognosis failed (LHR < 1.4 was chosen) and intervention conferred no benefit. Subsequently, it was incorporated into a more complex graphical version with observed to expected measurements to better correct for gestational age and provide a categorical expectation of survival (2). This was later used for the recent, larger multicenter Tracheal Occlusion To Accelerate Lung growth (TOTAL) trials (Chapter 6).

REFERENCES

1. Harrison MR, Keller RL, Hawgood SB, et al. A randomized trial of fetal endoscopic tracheal occlusion for severe fetal congenital diaphragmatic hernia. N Engl J Med. 2003;349:1916–24.
2. Jani J, Nicolaides KH, Keller RL, et al. Antenatal-CDH-Registry Group. Observed to expected lung area to head circumference ratio in the prediction of survival in fetuses with isolated diaphragmatic hernia. Ultrasound Obstet Gynecol. 2007;30(1):67–71. doi: 10.1002/uog.4052

A Randomized Trial of Prenatal versus Postnatal Repair of Myelomeningocele [Widely known as the Management of Myelomeningocele (MOMS) Trial]

NS Adzick, EA Thom, CY Spong, JW Brock, PK Burrows,
MP Johnson, LJ Howell, JA Farrell, ME Dabrowiak, LN Sutton,
N Gupta, NB Tulipan, ME D'Alton, and DL Farmer

New England Journal of Medicine 2011; 364(11): 993–1004.
Citations: n = 1,330

ABSTRACT

This was a randomized trial of prenatal repair of myelomeningocele (the most common form of spina bifida) with the standard postnatal repair with the hypothesis that there would be improved neurologic function.

Methods: Eligible women recruited from three American fetal medicine centers either underwent prenatal surgery before 26 weeks of gestation or standard postnatal repair. There were two primary outcomes: a composite of fetal or neonatal death or the need for placement of a cerebrospinal fluid shunt by the age of 12 months and a composite of mental development and motor function at 30 months.

Results: The trial was stopped for efficacy of prenatal surgery after the recruitment of 183 of a planned 200 patients. The report is based on results in 158 patients whose children were evaluated at 12 months. The first primary outcome occurred in 68% of the infants in the prenatal-surgery group and in 98% of those in the postnatal-surgery group (relative risk, 0.70; 97.7% confidence interval [CI], 0.58 to 0.84; P < 0.001). Actual rates of shunt placement were 40% in the prenatal-surgery group and 82% in the postnatal-surgery group (relative risk, 0.48; 97.7% CI, 0.36 to 0.64; P < 0.001). Prenatal surgery also resulted in improvement in the composite score for mental development and motor function at 30 months (P = 0.007) and in improvement in several secondary outcomes, including hindbrain herniation by 12 months and ambulation by 30 months. However, prenatal surgery was associated with an increased risk of preterm delivery and uterine dehiscence at delivery.

DOI: 10.1201/9781003341901-5

Conclusions: Prenatal surgery for myelomeningocele reduced the need for shunting and improved motor outcomes at 30 months but was associated with maternal and fetal risks.

COMMENTARY (MARK DAVENPORT)

Fetal surgery has its origins in the Fetal Treatment Center in San Francisco set up by Michael Harrison in the late 1980s. Its main object at that time was to try to improve outcomes of infants with congenital diaphragmatic hernias. A whole series of reports using a variety of interventions emanated from there, culminating in a randomized controlled trial published in 2003 (1). However, this showed no difference from conventionally treated infants in the postnatal period, leading to virtual abandonment of the programme.

The first human prenatal myelomeningocele repairs were first reported in 1998 from Children's Hospital of Philadelphia (2) and Nashville (3). This work and later reports seemed to show improvements in neurological outcomes albeit still with the hazards of preterm labour and even fetal demise. The MOMS trial (great title!) was carried out in three centres in Philadelphia, Nashville and San Francisco with surgeons using the same techniques and protocols.

Predictably, the mean gestational age in the fetal intervention group was 34.1 weeks (vs 37.3 weeks), and 13% (vs 0%) were delivered before 30 weeks of gestation. There were four deaths, two in each arm: in the fetal intervention group at 23–24 weeks gestation, and in the standard group postnatally due to severe hindbrain herniation.

As to the first primary outcome, there was big reduction in the need for cerebrospinal fluid (CSF) shunting (40% vs 82%) by 12 months, and it increased the proportion who had no evidence of hindbrain herniation well (36% vs 4%). Similarly, there was a large difference in their chosen composite score evaluating neuromuscular and developmental aspects.

Follow-up studies (4) focussing on more meaningful outcomes relevant to daily life showed that almost twice as many members of the fetal intervention group achieved independent walking (45% vs 24%), though those proportions reduced when looked at later when the groups were of school age (29% vs 11% – walking without aids). Urological outcomes at school age were somewhat better with reduced need for clean intermittent catheterisation (62% vs 87%), a higher proportion with voluntary voiding (24% vs 4%) but interestingly no significant differences in objective urodynamics or urological ultrasound assessments (5).

This trial encouraged the provision of fetal intervention for this condition in many centres worldwide, though it is still a formidable undertaking. It also implies relocation of the family for the duration of the pregnancy and without guarantee of a normal child at the end.

REFERENCES

1. Harrison MR, Keller RL, Hawgood SB, et al. A randomized trial of fetal endoscopic tracheal occlusion for severe fetal congenital diaphragmatic hernia. N Engl J Med. 2003;349(20):1916–24. doi: 10.1056/NEJMoa035005
2. Adzick NS, Sutton LN, Cromblehome TN, Flake AW. Successful fetal surgery for spina bifida. Lancet. 1998;352:1675–76.
3. Tulipan N, Hernanz-Schulman M, Bruner JP. Reduced hindbrain herniation after intrauterine myelomeningocele repair: A report of four cases. Pediatr Neurosurg. 1998;29(5):274–78. doi: 10.1159/000028735
4. Houtrow AJ, Thom EA, Fletcher JM, et al. Prenatal repair of myelomeningocele and school-age functional outcomes. Pediatrics. 2020;145(2):e20191544. doi: 10.1542/peds.2019-1544
5. Brock JW 3rd, Thomas JC, Baskin LS, et al. Effect of prenatal repair of myelomeningocele on urological outcomes at school age. J Urol. 2019;202(4):812–18. doi: 10.1097/JU.0000000000000334

CHAPTER 6

Randomized Trial of Fetal Surgery for Severe Left Diaphragmatic Hernia (Known as the TOTAL Trial)

Jan A Deprest, Kypros H Nicolaides, Alexandra Benachi, Eduard Gratacos, et al. TOTAL Trial for Severe Hypoplasia Investigators

New England Journal of Medicine 2021 July 8; 385(2):107–118.
Citations: $n = 139$

ABSTRACT

Observational studies have shown that fetoscopic endoluminal tracheal occlusion (FETO) has been associated with increased survival amongst infants with severe pulmonary hypoplasia due to isolated congenital diaphragmatic hernia (CDH) on the left side, but data from randomized trials are lacking.

Methods: The tracheal occlusion to accelerate lung growth (TOTAL) trial was an open-label multicentre ($n = 10$) randomized trial of FETO in fetuses with severe left-sided CDH. Severity was defined by and observed to the expected lung-to-head ratio that predicted survivals of <25%, with FETO initiated at 27 to 29 weeks of gestation. Primary outcome was infant survival to discharge from the neonatal intensive care unit.

Results: The trial was stopped early when a difference emerged after 80 women were recruited. In the FETO group, 16/40 (40%) of infants survived, as compared with 6/40 (15%) in the expectant care group (relative risk, 2.67; 95% confidence interval [CI], 1.22 to 6.11; two-sided P = 0.009). This difference persisted to survival at six months of age. As anticipated, the incidence of preterm rupture of membranes was higher in the FETO group (47% vs 11%; relative risk, 4.51; 95% CI, 1.83 to 11.9), as was the incidence of preterm birth (75% vs 29%; relative risk, 2.59; 95% CI, 1.59 to 4.52).

There was one neonatal death that occurred after emergency delivery for placental laceration from fetoscopic balloon removal, and one neonatal death occurred because of failed balloon removal.

Amongst the secondary outcomes examined, there was less use of extracorporeal membrane oxygenation (ECMO) (2/40 (5%) vs 11/38 (29%)).

DOI: 10.1201/9781003341901-6

Conclusions: FETO offers improved survival in fetuses who have left-sided CDH and severe lung hypoplasia.

COMMENTARY (MARK DAVENPORT)

Background

The concept of tracheal occlusion for severe diaphragmatic hernias had been developed in Michael Harrison's Fetal Treatment Center in San Francisco in the 1990s. This concept mimicked a natural experiment, in that congenital laryngeal atresia causes overdevelopment and hyperplasia of the fetal lungs with inversion of the diaphragms. Various ways were investigated of replicating this including direct application of surgical clips to the exposed fetal trachea and ultimately placing an expanding balloon within the lumen. This culminated in an actual randomized trial (1) which was stopped before completion, as there proved to be no difference in outcome between the fetal intervention arm and those allowed to be delivered with conventional management. So, progress in the USA in this field stopped. However, in Leuven, Belgium, a trained obstetrician and fetal medicine specialist (as opposed to a paediatric surgeon), Jan Deprest, reinvestigated its potential. He used a much less invasive approach of fetoscopy via a single 3 mm port and a detachable balloon derived from an embolectomy catheter used in vascular intervention. He later introduced the concept of balloon removal prior to delivery (usually by a second fetoscopy). This technique was then applied progressively in European centres in London and Barcelona and then exported back to North America.

This trial was designed to combat scepticism primarily in North American centres over the efficacy of FETO. The aforementioned San Francisco trial had been followed by a small Brazilian trial (2), but this was much larger and more comprehensive. Nevertheless, it took a long time to recruit the numbers (95 were randomized over almost 10 years), and these represented a fairly small proportion of the 1,314 women with CDH fetuses seen during the period. The trial emphasised that the known problems of premature birth were still present with FETO infants (75% vs 39%). There was less use of ECMO in the FETO group, and the other manifestations of CDH (e.g., pulmonary hypertension) appeared similar in the survivors.

There was also a parallel trial, published in the same issue of *The New England Journal of Medicine* (3), looking at FETO in a group of fetuses with moderate lung hypoplasia, where the balloon was inserted later (30–32 weeks' gestation). This recruited much higher numbers ($n = 196$ women) with survival in the FETO group being greater (62/98 (63%) vs 49/98 (50%)) but of borderline statistical significance (relative risk, 1.27; 95% confidence interval [CI], 0.99 to 1.63; two-sided $P = 0.06$). Interestingly, the incidence of premature birth, though still higher (44% vs 12%), was lower than in the severe hypoplasia group with earlier FETO insertion.

REFERENCES

1. Harrison MR, Keller RL, Hawgood SB, et al. A randomized trial of fetal endoscopic tracheal occlusion for severe fetal congenital diaphragmatic hernia. N Engl J Med. 2003;349:1916–24.
2. Ruano R, Yoshisaki CT, da Silva MM, et al. A randomized controlled trial of fetal endoscopic tracheal occlusion versus postnatal management of severe isolated congenital diaphragmatic hernia. Ultrasound Obstet Gynecol. 2012;39:20–27.
3. Deprest JA, Benachi A, Gratacos E, et al. TOTAL Trial for Moderate Hypoplasia Investigators. Randomized trial of fetal surgery for moderate left diaphragmatic hernia. N Engl J Med. 2021;385(2):119–29. doi: 10.1056/NEJMoa2026983

Percutaneous Vesicoamniotic Shunting versus Conservative Management for Fetal Lower Urinary Tract Obstruction (PLUTO): A Randomised Trial

Rachel K Morris, Gemma L Malin, Elisabeth Quinlan-Jones,
Lee J Middleton, Karla Hemming, Danielle Burke, Jane P Daniels,
Khalid S Khan, Jon Deeks, and Mark D Kilby

Lancet 2013; 382: 1496–506
Citations: *n* = 250

ABSTRACT

PLUTO was an international, multicentre randomized control trial that aimed at testing improved survival and renal outcomes in infant with lower urinary tract obstruction (LUTO) that had undergone fetal vesicoamniotic shunt (VAS) in comparison to expectant management.

Methods: *Study cohort:* Women with singleton male pregnancies complicated by LUTO.

Randomisation: Twenty-one fetal medicine units in the United Kingdom, Ireland and the Netherlands participated and were recruited to the trial between October 2006 to October 2010.

Intervention: Ultrasound (USS) guided percutaneous insertion of a vesicoamniotic shunt within seven days of randomisation.

Primary outcome: Survival at 28 days after birth.

Secondary outcomes: Survival at one and two years, and renal function at 28 days, one year and two years.

Results: 144 eligible pregnancies were screened in all participating centres, 68 (47%) opted for termination of pregnancy (TOP) and 45 (31%) joined the LUTO registry but did not consent for the trial. Thirty-one (22%) were recruited from 7 (33%) of the 21 participating centres; 16 were randomized to the VAS arm and 15 to the conservative

DOI: 10.1201/9781003341901-7

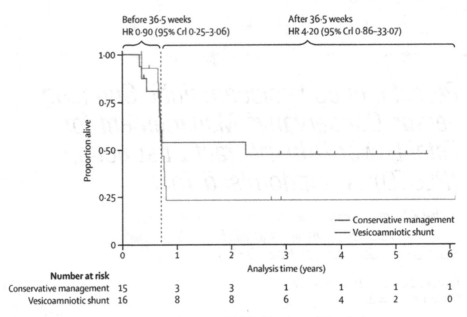

Figure 7.1   Kaplan–Meier Survival Curves in PLUTO. (Courtesy of Elsevier.)

management arm. Three of the 16 pregnancies in the intervention arm did not receive a VAS, and two of the 15 in the conservative management arm had shunting.

Overall, 15 fetuses recruited in the trial underwent a VAS. There were five TOPs, three in the intervention arm, two of which were a treatment-related complication, and two in the conservative arm. There was one fetal demise reported in each study arm, and the one in the intervention group was treatment related. There were 24 live births (77.4%) overall, 12 in each trial group (Figure 7.1).

Median gestational age at LUTO diagnosis was 21 weeks (interquartile range [IQR], 18–22). A high proportion of fetuses had a second-trimester oligohydramnios (amniotic fluid is <5th centile for gestational age); 10/16 (63%) in the shunt group and 9/15 (60%) in the conservative group. Gestational age at delivery was comparable between the two groups (shunt 34.6 weeks [IQR 33.4–37.2 vs 36.4 weeks [IQR 34.5–37.4]). The mean birth weight in the two groups was 2.8 kg. Six neonates in the intervention and seven in the conservative group required ventilation support after birth. Treatment for renal impairment occurred in four infants in the intervention group and three in the conservative group.

Twelve neonatal deaths due to pulmonary hypoplasia ensued; 11 occurred within the first 24 h after birth, and the last at 3 days of age. A further two deaths occurred by the first year, one in each trial arm. In an intention to treat analysis, eight (8/16; 50%) infants in the shunt group and four (4/15; 27%) infants in the conservative management group survived to 28 days (RR = 1·88, CI [0·71–4·96]; p = 0·27). Survival at one and two years was similar, 7/16 in the intervention group and 3/15 in the conservative management group (RR = 2·19, CI [0·69–6·94]; p = 0·25).

Renal impairment at 28 days was observed in 6/8 in the intervention group and 4/4 in the conservative management group. Only two infants from the intervention group did not have renal impairment at one-year follow-up. By two years, moderate renal impairment was observed in 5/7 in the intervention group and 2/3 in the conservative group, while the last child in this group had an end-stage renal failure.

The final diagnosis leading to LUTO was confirmed in 18/31 cases. Of the 24 live births, nine had posterior urethral valves (five in the VAS group and four in the conservative group), five had urethral atresia (four in the VAS group and one in the conservative group) and one case of urethral syrinx that caused obstruction (in the conservative group). All infants with posterior urethral valves underwent valve ablation within six weeks of birth, and all those with urethral atresia had a vesicostomy formed.

Conclusion
Fetuses with LUTO undergoing VAS seemed to have higher survival. Yet the results of this trial suggest that, irrespective of intervention, the chance of infants surviving with normal renal function is very low.

COMMENTARY (BASHAR ALDEIRI)

The PLUTO trial, conceived and led from Birmingham, UK, was unique in the sense that it was the very first randomized trial of fetal intervention for a urological disease. Unfortunately, poor recruitment led to early trial closure with only a fifth of the recruitment target over four years. A great opportunity was missed as, the authors have concluded (1); clinical trials in paediatric surgery are exceptionally difficult to organise and coordinate and extremely expensive to run, and the PLUTO trial was a breviary of all these barriers in paediatric research.

The trial did provide some valuable information for clinicians and families of fetuses with LUTO. This was perhaps not just the survival data but the expectations if the child were actually to survive. Only one of the surviving children had normal renal function at two years. There was an element of preselection in that chosen fetuses tended to have the worse outcomes. Over half had significant oligohydramnios, and a diagnosis of urethral atresia was made in seven of 18 with a confirmed final diagnosis. There is now consensus that the presence of anhydramnios early in the second trimester results in a fetal mortality rate close to 100%, and untreated fetal LUTO with an early onset (first or early second trimester of pregnancy) can lead to death in up to 80% of fetuses (2). Yet, there is an argument nowadays that VAS performed early in the second trimester for LUTO provides better outcomes. A recent study demonstrated a higher proportion of normal renal function and reduced incidence of pulmonary hypoplasia in the surviving infants who had a VAS before the completion of 16 weeks' gestation (3). Nevertheless, this study was not randomized or controlled.

For the time being, the PLUTO trial and other cohort studies suggest that expectant parents of fetuses with LUTO should be prepared to deal with substantial lifelong comorbidity in surviving children.

REFERENCES

1. Morris RK, Daniels J, Deeks J, Field D, Kilby MD. The challenges of interventional trials in fetal therapy. Arch Dis Child Fetal Neonatal Ed. 2014;99(6):F448–50.
2. Capone V, Persico N, Berrettini A, Decramer S, et al. Definition, diagnosis and management of fetal lower urinary tract obstruction: consensus of the ERKNet CAKUT-Obstructive Uropathy Work Group. Nat Rev Urol. 2022;19(5):295–303.
3. Kohl T, Fimmers R, Axt-Fliedner R, Degenhardt J, Brückmann M. Vesico-amniotic shunt insertion prior to the completion of 16 weeks results in improved preservation of renal function in surviving fetuses with isolated severe lower urinary tract obstruction (LUTO). J Pediatr Urol. 2022;18(2):116–26.

CHAPTER 8

Thoracoscopic Repair of Esophageal Atresia and Tracheoesophageal Fistula: A Multi-Institutional Analysis

George W Holcomb III, Steven S Rothenberg, Klaas MA Bax,
Marcelo Martinez-Ferro, Craig T Albanese, Daniel J Ostlie,
David C van Der Zee, and CK Yeung

Annals of Surgery 242: 422–430, 2005
Citations: $n = 240$

ABSTRACT

Objectives: A multi-institutional, multinational review of the largest experience to date with a thoracoscopic approach to esophageal atresia.

Methods: Retrospective review from six centres of 104 newborns with esophageal atresia (EA)/tracheoesophageal fistula (TEF). Newborns with EA without a distal TEF or those with an isolated TEF without EA were excluded.

Results: In these 104 patients, the mean age at operation was 1.2 days (standard deviation [SD] 1.1), the mean weight was 2.6 kg (SD 0.5), the mean operative time was 130 minutes (SD 55.5), the mean days of mechanical ventilation were 3.6 (SD 5.8), and the mean days of total hospitalisation were 18 (SD 18.6). Five operations (4.8%) were converted to an open thoracotomy, and one was staged due to a long gap between the two esophageal segments. Twelve infants (11.5%) developed an early leak or stricture at the anastomosis, and 33 (31.7%) required esophageal dilatation at least once. Twenty-five newborns (24%) later required a laparoscopic fundoplication. A recurrent TEF developed in two infants (1.9%).

A number of other operations were required in these patients, including imperforate anus repair in 10 patients ($n = 7$ high, $n = 3$ low), aortopexy ($n = 7$), laparoscopic duodenal atresia repair ($n = 4$) and various major cardiac operations ($n = 5$). Three patients died, one related to the EA/TEF on the 20th postoperative day.

Conclusions: Thoracoscopic repair of EA/TEF represents a natural evolution in the operative correction of this complicated congenital anomaly and can be safely performed by experienced endoscopic surgeons. The results presented are comparable to previous reports approaching this through a thoracotomy. Based on

DOI: 10.1201/9781003341901-8

the associated musculoskeletal problems following thoracotomy, there will likely be long-term benefits for babies with this anomaly undergoing the thoracoscopic repair.

COMMENTARY (GEORGE 'WHIT' HOLCOMB III)

I remember the idea behind this paper as if it were yesterday. One must remember the background behind this paper. Minimally invasive surgery was really in its infancy, especially compared to now, when Steve Rothenberg and Thom Lobe performed the first thoracoscopic repair of EA without a TEF while at the International Pediatric Endosurgery Group (IPEG) meeting in Berlin in 1999. A 3.4 kg baby had undergone serial bougienage until the two esophageal segments were close enough to attempt the repair. A year later, Steve reported the first thoracoscopic repair of EA/TEF in a newborn as part of his Presidential Address at the 2000 IPEG meeting. So, our group at Children's Mercy Hospital in Kansas City, and other experienced minimally invasive surgery (MIS) surgeons, began to utilize this approach on selected babies.

In the early 2000s, there were only a few scattered case reports that described an individual surgeon's experience with thoracoscopic repair of EA/TEF. I knew Steve had performed a number of these operations in the few years following his initial report and had reported his initial case series in 2002. I also knew all the authors were doing these operations as well, so I thought it would be good if all of us could combine our experiences for this paper. First, I was surprised at the number of these operations ($n = 104$) our author group had performed between 2000 and 2004. Second, I was also very surprised at how good the results were (see the preceding abstract for details). Twelve infants (11.5%) developed an early leak or stricture at the anastomosis, and 33 (31.7%) required esophageal dilatation at least once. Five operations (4.8%) were converted to an open thoracotomy. Also, in this paper, we compared our thoracoscopic experience for EA/TEF with the published experience with the open approach from several large centers, and our data compared very favorably with these large open series.

I also knew Steve was probably too busy to take the lead on this paper, so I organized the effort. However, I thought Steve should receive his due credit for his pioneering efforts, so I had him present the paper at the 2005 meeting of the American Surgical Association meeting. I also figured I knew the data better than anyone else as the first author on the paper, so I was the discussant as I thought some of the questions would focus on the data and not as much on the technique. After the presentation, the questions came from a legendary group of pediatric surgeons: Jim O'Neill, Jud Randolph, John Foker and Marshall Schwartz.

All in all, it was a very well-received presentation and subsequent publication. I give credit to all the authors for their pioneering efforts on their respective continents for being excellent surgeons and innovators.

COMMENTARY (MARK DAVENPORT)

The first thoracoscopic repair of an oesophageal atresia had been reported only a few years before (1999), but this had stimulated action in a number of pioneering centres, well represented here in the author list from the American Midwest, Argentina, the Netherlands and Hong Kong. Though the approach was the same the actual techniques used varied considerably with different ways of closing the fistula (clips, ligation), anastomotic suture material (PDS™, Vicryl™, silk, etc.) and even knot tying (evenly divided between extracorporeal and intracorporeal) varied. There were three deaths, mostly related to coincident cardiac disease, and the complications were as one might expect, aside from perhaps a higher stricture rate of 32%. The paper contrasts their experience with published open series, though some were somewhat dated, even for 2005.

This paper showed that thoracoscopy could be a valid and safe alternative to the open procedure (in the hands of experts), though the main perceived advantage (preservation of chest wall integrity) was never and probably will never be evaluated.

At the conclusion, they make a plea for a randomized trial, though of course this too will never happen. In the intervening years, despite this and other papers, open repairs are still far more commonly performed. Why? Because an expert surgeon is required to perform this operation, and many cases are needed to build the necessary thoracoscopic competence and there are many parts of the world where such cases are uncommon and case-load/surgeon is low.

CHAPTER 9

Experience with 220 Consecutive Laparoscopic Nissen Fundoplications in Infants and Children

Steven S Rothenberg

Journal of Pediatric Surgery 1998; 33: 274–278.
Citations: $n = 163$

ABSTRACT

Background/purpose: Fundoplication for gastroesophageal reflux disease is a common procedure performed in infants and children. This report describes a four-year experience with 220 consecutive laparoscopic Nissen fundoplications.

Methods: Ages ranged from five days to 18 years and weight from 1.4 to 100 kg. The procedures were performed using a five-trocar technique and with 5 or 3.4 mm instruments depending on the size of the patient. Technique involved a full crural dissection, mobilisation of an adequate length intra-abdominal oesophagus, crural repair and a 1 to 4 cm-long 360° anterior fundal wrap secured with two to four sutures, including the anterior oesophageal wall.

Results: Two hundred and eighteen fundoplications were completed successfully. Age and weight at time of surgery ranged between five days to 18 years, and 1.4 to 110 kg, respectively. The main indication for surgery was gastro-oesophageal reflux disease (GERD) that did not respond to attempts (a course) of medical therapy. Only 27/220 (12%) were neurologically impaired, and 18/220 (8%) had severe oesophagitis or an oesophageal stricture on upper gastrointestinal (GI) endoscopy. A gastrostomy was placed in 143 cases (65%), and a concurrent pyloroplasty was performed in seven patients.

Average operative time dropped dramatically from 109 to 55 minutes for the first 30 cases compared with the last 30. Intraoperative and postoperative complication rates were 2.6% and 7.3%, respectively. Average time to discharge postfundoplication was 1.6 days. The follow-up period ranged between 3 and 53 months. Intraoperative complications occurred in three cases (one gastric and one oesophageal perforation and one left-sided pneumothorax). Postoperative dysphagia occurred in four cases (~ 2%), two of which required oesophageal dilatation. The wrap failure rate was 3.4%.

DOI: 10.1201/9781003341901-9

Conclusions: This study shows that although the learning curve for laparoscopic fundoplication may be steep, the procedure is safe and effective in the pediatric population. The clinical results are comparable to the traditional open fundoplication but with a significant decrease in morbidity and hospitalization.

COMMENTARY (STEVEN S ROTHENBERG)

In 1993, I presented a video at the annual meeting of American Pediatric Surgical Association (APSA) in Hilton Head, South Carolina, 'Laparoscopic Nissen Fundoplication and Percutaneous G-Tube Placement for the Management of GER: A New Technique in Children'. This had been one of the first laparoscopic fundoplications I had performed, and the video was met with a great deal of scepticism. 'I can do that operation through a 2 cm incision', 'it takes too long', 'it's not as good, as open', 'it doesn't work', 'there will be a high failure rate' and 'my scars are tiny and not an issue'.

Over the next four years, I worked hard to perfect the technique and collect prospective data on every patient that I performed the procedure on. In the interim, I presented the technique at IPEG, the Society of American Gastrointestinal and Endoscopic Surgeons (SAGES) and other forums where the reception was much more positive. I wanted to present the technique and the data at APSA because this was the major forum for North American pediatric surgeons and I thought it was important for the members to be exposed to this technique. I knew that because of the inherent bias against MIS at APSA that the data would have to be so overwhelming that the technique could not be questioned. I felt a series of over 200 patients over a five-year period by a single surgeon would be proof of the technique and the results. I was fortunate to be in a hospital where neonatology, pulmonology and gastroenterology felt severe reflux should be treated aggressively to prevent long-term pulmonary and GI complications, and thus I was able to collect a large number of cases over a relatively short period of time. The intraoperative complication rate was <3%, average operative time <1 hour, and average length of stay was <2 days. Not surprisingly, when presented at APSA, the discussion turned from the quality of the technique to the surgical indications, a tacit acknowledgement that a laparoscopic approach was superior to an open approach. I believe this paper helped establish laparoscopic Nissen fundoplication as the gold standard in children.

COMMENTARY (BASHAR ALDEIRI)

This was not just the largest paediatric Nissen fundoplication series of its time but perhaps the largest paediatric laparoscopic series of any kind. It does not come as a surprise that it is reported by a true pioneer in pediatric minimally invasive surgery, Steven S Rothenberg from the Rocky Mountain Children's Hospital, Denver, Colorado. He presented the paper at the 28th APSA Meeting in Florida, and reading through that meeting's discussion is sufficient to grasp how the paper was perceived as a landmark then though somewhat controversial, and perhaps it still is to this day.

The paper represented a school of thought that favoured an early surgical approach in infants and children with GERD. They saw the fundoplication as a curative operation with little adverse effects, and the feasibility to perform it in a minimally invasive fashion was a major bonus (1, 2). Yet, the main controversy this paper raised was the perhaps too-liberal use of fundoplication as a primary treatment for GERD. The series implies one laparoscopic fundoplication a week for four years with most patients (55%) being infants <10 kg. Many would probably echo Dr Denis King's comment during the 28th APSA meeting: 'The ability to do something is not an indication to do it'. The paper represents dedication and perseverance to prove feasibility and adequacy of minimally invasive surgery in children. It is also a clear demonstration of the importance of the learning curve when adopting a new approach even for established surgeons.

Certainly, in the intervening years, laparoscopic fundoplication has become the cliched 'gold standard' for surgical treatment of GERD in infants and children as it is in adults. Gastro-oesophageal reflux, however, is a physiological process in this age group, and regurgitation symptoms can be recorded in up to 70% of young infants – the possibility of overtreatment is high. So now, the lure of early fundoplication in the management of GERD in children seems to be fading (3). It clearly still has a role, though societal guidelines from both sides of the Atlantic (4) emphasise prolonged medical management much more, and a structured approach to diagnosis including increasing use of 24-hour multichannel manometry-impedance studies. Similarly, a stepwise surgical approach offers better overall care and is strongly advocated. Gastrostomy tube insertion as a first step can be equally as effective in some cases and is completely reversible. It also has the advantage of being able to be upgraded to transpyloric feeding using a wide array of commercially available devices (3). These have certainly changed the scene and are widely used with perhaps comparable outcomes to fundoplication overall (5–7). Several studies have shown a reduction of the rates of apnoea and bradycardia in neonates with GERD when using a transpyloric feeding regimen (5, 6).

Children with neurological disability and GERD are problematic and tend to have an unfavourable outcome and the highest failure rate of a fundoplication (8), though not of course in the Rothenberg paper. Also, the role of (Nissen) fundoplication is still controversial and has the most problems postoperatively. Most of these children are still on pharmacological anti-acid treatment (9), and the possibility of long-term failure, and indeed mortality, is high. Dissatisfaction has led to some some centers advocating for the fairly aggressive alternative of esophagogastric dissociation because of the perceived ineffectiveness of a Nissen in controlling GERD (10).

REFERENCES

1. Pacilli M, Eaton S, McHoney M, Kiely EM, et al. Four year follow-up of a randomised controlled trial comparing open and laparoscopic Nissen fundoplication in children. Arch Dis Child. 2014;99(6):516–21.

2. Kubiak R, Spitz L, Kiely EM, Drake D, Pierro A. Effectiveness of fundoplication in early infancy. J Pediatr Surg. 1999;34(2):295–99.
3. Khan FA, Nestor K, Hashmi A, Islam S. To wrap or not? Utility of anti-reflux procedure in infants needing gastrostomy tubes. Front Pediatr. 2022;10:855156.
4. Rosen R, Vandenplas Y, Singendonk M, Cabana M, et al. Pediatric gastroesophageal reflux clinical practice guidelines: joint recommendations of the NASPGHN and the ESPGHAN. J Pediatr Gastroenterol Nutr. 2018;66:516–54.
5. Malcolm WF, Smith PB, Mears S, Goldberg RN, Cotten CM. Transpyloric tube feeding in very low birthweight infants with suspected gastroesophageal reflux: impact on apnea and bradycardia. J Perinatol. 2009;29:372–75.
6. Srivastava R, Downey EC, O'Gorman M, Feola P, et al. Impact of fundoplication versus gastrojejunal feeding tubes on mortality and in preventing aspiration pneumonia in young children with neurologic impairment who have gastroesophageal reflux disease. Pediatrics. 2009;123(1):338–45.
7. Barnhart DC, Hall M, Mahant S, Goldin AB, et al. Effectiveness of fundoplication at the time of gastrostomy in infants with neurological impairment. JAMA Pediatr. 2013;167:911–18.
8. Capito C, Leclair M-D, Piloquet H, Plattner V, Heloury Y, Podevin G. Long-term outcome of laparoscopic Nissen-Rossetti fundoplication for neurologically impaired and normal children. Surg Endosc. 2008;22(4):875–80.
9. Lee SL, Sydorak RM, Chiu VY, Hsu J-W, et al. Long-term antireflux medication use following pediatric Nissen fundoplication. Arch Surg. 2008;143:873–76.
10. Lansdale N, McNiff M, Morecroft J, Kauffmann L, Morabito A. Long-term and "patient-reported" outcomes of total esophagogastric dissociation versus laparoscopic fundoplication for gastroesophageal reflux disease in the severely neurodisabled child. J Pediatr Surg. 2015;50:1828–32.

CHAPTER 10

Open versus Laparoscopic Pyloromyotomy for Pyloric Stenosis: A Prospective, Randomized Trial

Shawn St Peter, George W Holcomb III, Casey Calkins, J Patrick Murphy, et al.

Annals of Surgery 2006; 244: 363–370.
Citations: *n* = 173

ABSTRACT

Background: Pyloric stenosis, the most common surgical condition of infants, is treated by longitudinal myotomy of the pylorus. Comparative studies to date between open and laparoscopic pyloromyotomy have been retrospective and report conflicting results. To scientifically compare the two techniques, we conducted the first large prospective, randomized trial between the two approaches.

Methods: Ultrasound-proven pyloric stenosis were randomized to either open or laparoscopic pyloromyotomy. Postoperative pain management, feeding schedule and discharge criteria were identical for both groups. Operating time, postoperative emesis, analgesia requirements, time to full feeding, length of hospitalisation after operation and complications were compared.

Results: From April 2003 through March 2006, 200 patients were enrolled in the study. There were no significant differences in operating time, time to full feeding or length of stay. There were significantly fewer number of emesis episodes and doses of analgesia given in the laparoscopic group. One mucosal perforation and one incisional hernia occurred in the open group. Late in the study, one patient in the laparoscopic group was converted to the open operation. A wound infection occurred in four of the open patients compared with two of the laparoscopic patients (*P* = 0.68).

Conclusions: There is no difference in operating time or length of recovery between open and laparoscopic pyloromyotomy. However, the laparoscopic approach results in less postoperative pain and reduced postoperative emesis. In addition, there were fewer complications in the laparoscopic group. Finally, patients approached laparoscopically will likely display superior cosmetic outcomes with long-term follow-up.

COMMENTARY (JOE DAVIDSON)

Although Rammstedt's procedure has been performed as described for many years since its introduction, leading to pyloric stenosis being a completely survivable

DOI: 10.1201/9781003341901-10

condition, focus has now shifted towards improving the quality of the surgical care provided. Adrian Bianchi described in 1986 (1) the use of a circumumbilical incision to access pyloric stenosis, which provides the same visualization as a right-upper quadrant incision with almost imperceptible scarring. This incision has now become the standard of care for many neonatal open procedures in many centres but noticeably not in the centre in this trial, which still used the 'old-fashioned' right-upper quadrant incision. The first laparoscopic pyloromyotomy was published in 1991 by Alain et al. from Limoges, France (2), and since that time the practice has been favoured by many surgeons in the absence of direct comparative evidence.

This single-centre randomized trial compared either a standardised laparoscopic pyloromyotomy (using knife and spreader) or an open pyloromyotomy (typically right-upper quadrant muscle cutting). Since the most important outcomes were rare (incomplete myotomy and mucosal perforation) and therefore not feasible to power the study, the authors elected to use a minimum recruitment that was powered to detect differences in operative time (60 per arm) and then went beyond this to achieve better resolution for the rarer events (100 per arm). They showed nearly identical outcomes for operative time, with a reduced but not statistically significant reduction in time to feeds and length of stay in the laparoscopic group. There were significant differences favouring the laparoscopic approach regarding postoperative emesis and for the nurse-assessed and administered analgesia postoperatively (a recognised subjective outcome measure). Interestingly, these differences were replicated very closely in a similarly sized multicentre trial by Hall et al. published a few years later (3).

To date there have been seven randomized controlled trials (RCTs), last reviewed in 2022 (4) trying to answer this question – 'which is better?' – involving 720 patients (open procedures, $n = 357$ and laparoscopic procedures, $n = 363$) with a variety of primary endpoints. Essentially, meta-analysis suggests no real difference in mucosal perforation rates but a non-significant risk of incomplete pyloromyotomy in the laparoscopic group (RR 7.37 [0.92–59.11]). Wound infection, seromas rates etc. were similar. Length of stay and time to full feeds were nonsignificantly shorter after laparoscopic pyloromyotomy.

This study merits landmark status given that it is an RCT on a common problem – albeit 15 years after the procedure in question was first described – and is another one of a series from the American Midwest (Kansas City). The clinical relevance of its primary outcome (operative time) could be questioned, but it undoubtedly established the validity of the laparoscopic alternative.

REFERENCES

1. Tan KC, Bianchi A. Circumumbilical incision for pyloromyotomy. Br J Surg. 1986;73:399.
2. Alain JL, Grousseau D, Terrier G. Extramucosal pyloromyotomy by laparoscopy. J Pediatr Surg. 1991;26:1191–1119.

3. Hall NJ, Pacilli M, Eaton S, Reblock K, et al. Recovery after open versus laparoscopic pyloromyotomy for pyloric stenosis: a double-blind multicentre randomised controlled trial. Lancet. 2009;373:390–398.
4. Lunger F, Staerkle RF, Muff JL, Fink L, et al. Open versus laparoscopic pyloromyotomy for pyloric stenosis-a systematic review and meta-analysis. J Surg Res. 2022;274:1–8.

CHAPTER 11

Congenital Intestinal Atresia; Observations on Its Origin

Jannie H Louw and Christiaan N Barnard

Lancet. 1955 Nov 19; 269(6899):1065–1067.
Citations: $n = 402$

ABSTRACT

This is an exceptional paper, Figure 11.1 detailing the journey from clinical observation to experimental confirmation. The senior author (Jannie Louw) notes that during a visit to the wards at Great Ormond Street Hospital, London, where he reviewed cases of intestinal atresia, he noted that midgut atresias could often be characterised by blind ends and a 'V-shaped' gap in the mesentery. Some showed thrombosis in the vessels while others had clear evidence of some local event such as a localised volvulus or intussusception. They also quoted the work of Laufman et al. published in 1949 (1), who showed that devascularised, sterilised loops of bowel that were left within the peritoneal cavity of dogs simply converted into fibrous bands or indeed disappeared.

Christian Barnard, at this point in his career a surgical registrar, did the actual experiments on puppies *in utero*. This involved ligating the blood supply to a segment of small intestine. After many failures, he managed to get two to survive beyond the day of intervention itself, at three and 12 days. At postmortem, he found that the proximal ends of the intestine were both blind-ending and obstructed; in the first there was a necrotic segment in the process of disintegration, while in the second the two ends were joined by a fibrous cord with a gap in the mesentery. The pathology they attributed to a 'vascular accident'.

In the discussion, they advocated resection of the distal obstructed bowel found in intestinal atresias on the grounds that its blood supply may already be compromised.

CONGENITAL INTESTINAL ATRESIA
OBSERVATIONS ON ITS ORIGIN

J. H. LOUW   C. N. BARNARD
M.B., Ch.M. Cape Town   M.D. Cape Town
PROFESSOR OF SURGERY   SURGICAL REGISTRAR
DEPARTMENT OF SURGERY, UNIVERSITY OF CAPE TOWN

Figure 11.1 Courtesy of Elsevier.

DOI: 10.1201/9781003341901-11

Further, they remarked that this policy had already been adopted at Great Ormond Street with a consequent reduction in mortality from 69% to 33%.

There is a follow-up paper (2) with further descriptions, but finding a copy is difficult.

IMPACT (MARK DAVENPORT)

This has become the accepted theory for the genesis of small bowel atresia. The older one, enunciated by Tandler in 1912 (3), of failure of recanalisation of the lumen is still holding sway for duodenal atresia. Nevertheless, it is still difficult to discern what actually causes the vascular accident, as most atresia don't show a local volvulus, etc. There is circumstantial evidence of an association of intestinal atresia and maternal use of vasoconstrictive substances such as ergotamine tartrate, cocaine, amphetamine and pseudoephedrine. Indeed, smoking and thereby nicotine exposure are more common in such pregnancies (4).

Jannie Louw (1915–1992) is now regarded as the father of South African paediatric surgery and was the chief at Red Cross Children's Hospital in Cape Town. Christiaan Barnard (1922–2001) flew even higher, becoming an internationally-renowned cardiac surgeon at Groote Schuur Hospital in the same city. In December 1967, he led the team that performed the world's first successful heart transplant – the grateful recipient being a man named Louis Washkansky.

REFERENCES

1. Laufman, H., Martin, W. B., Method, H., Tuel, S. W., Harding, H. Arch. Surg. 1949; 59, 550.
2. Barnard CN, Louw JH. The genesis of intestinal atresia. Minn Med. 1956;39(11):745.
3. Tandler J. Zur entwicklungsgeschichte des menschlichen duodenum in fruhen embryonalstadien. Morphol Jahrb. 1912;29:187–216.
4. Sabbatini S, Ganji N, Chusilp S, Balsamo F, Li B, Pierro A. Intestinal atresia and necrotizing enterocolitis: Embryology and anatomy. Semin Pediatr Surg. 2022;31(6):151234.

CHAPTER 12

Oesophageal Atresia: At-Risk Groups for the 1990s

Lewis Spitz, Edward M Kiely, James A Morecroft, and David P Drake

Journal of Pediatric Surgery 1994; 29: 723–725.
Citations: n = 265

ABSTRACT

The authors analysed the outcome for 357 infants with oesophageal atresia and 15 with H-type tracheoesophageal fistula treated from 1980 through 1992 (Figure 12.1). Survival according to Waterston risk categories was 99% for group A, 95% for group B and 71% for group C.

Presently, with optimal management, virtually all infants in groups A and B should survive. When examining the risk factors in the infants who died, two criteria were found to be important predictors of outcome: birth weight of < 1,500 g and the

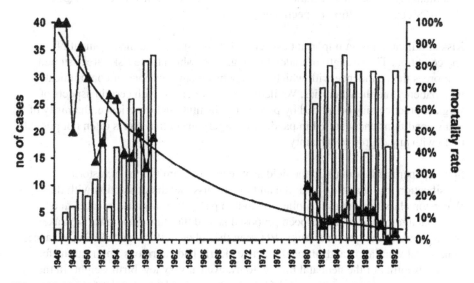

Figure 12.1 Mortality for cases of oesophageal atresia at Great Ormond Street Hospital: Waterston and Spitz compared.

DOI: 10.1201/9781003341901-12

presence of major congenital cardiac disease. Therefore, a new classification for predicting outcome in oesophageal atresia is proposed:

- Group I: birth weight ≥ 1,500 g, without major cardiac disease, survival 97% (283 of 293).
- Group II: birth weight < 1,500 g, or major cardiac disease, survival 59% (41 of 70).
- Group III: birth weight < 1,500 g, and major cardiac disease, survival 22% (2 of 9).

COMMENTARY (JOE DAVIDSON)

This was the largest reported series of oesophageal atresia (OA) at the time of its publication and still remains one of the largest to date.

It updated the preexisting Waterston classification (also from Great Ormond Street Hospital, London) published in 1962 (1). This pioneered risk stratification into (i) birth weight (two thresholds of 4 lb and 5.5 lb (1,800 and 2,500 g); (ii) additional anomalies (defined as mild or moderate if affecting the skeleton or cardiac without circulatory compromise – ASD or small PDA; or severe if a major cardiac anomaly or renal or intestinal atresia); and (iii) postoperative pneumonia (defined as moderate or severe), which represented a surrogate for anastomotic breakdown. Waterston Group A defined infants > 2,500 g with no anomalies and no pneumonia as having an excellent prognosis, while group B were infants 2,500–1,800 g or those with moderate pneumonia *and* an associated anomaly, while Group C were < 1,800 g *or* had severe pneumonia and a severe congenital anomaly. The survival rates were 36/38 (95%), 29/43 (68%) and 2/32 (6%) respectively.

Risk stratification is an important aspect in the assessment and management of any condition. The strength of understanding, upon which these risks are assumed, reinforces the confidence with which we may make our decisions or communicate with patients and their families. While the risks associated with certain aspects of surgical practice may be guided by personal or institutional experience, the rarity of many conditions encountered in paediatric surgery mean that this is often not possible to do with any degree of certainty.

Spitz's paper is a landmark in the field as it recognises limitations of historic classification in a changing field: the authors discuss the 'dissatisfaction with the Waterston classification as it applies to modern paediatric surgical practice' and state that alternatives that had been proposed lacked the statistical power to make conclusions of equivalent certainty. Between the cohorts (1950s and 1980s), advances in neonatal ventilation and surgical practice clearly had enormous implications for the survivability of the neonatal thoracotomy, even at very low birth weight. In the lowest birth weight group (those < 1,500 g birth weight) the survival rate is greater than 60%. The authors found the most relevant additional determinant of survival to be major cardiac disease, defined as a lesion requiring surgical correction or treatment of cardiac failure.

Spitz concludes his paper 'with continuing advances … even higher survival rates can be expected for infants with OA. In the meantime, we believe the proposed classification will be useful to give parents a realistic prognosis and to compare results.' Indeed, Spitz's risk scoring is the most commonly used system even today; several papers in recent years have attempted to update or modify the score further but deviate little from the original definitions (2). There has even been another reevaluation from the team at Great Ormond Street (3) highlighting the relative diminution in the influence of the birth weight on mortality.

REFERENCES

1. Waterston DJ, Bonham Carter RE, Aberdeen E. Oesophageal atresia: trachea-oesophageal fistula. A study of survival in 218 infants. Lancet. 1962;279:819–22.
2. Okamoto T, Takamizawa S, Arai H, Bitoh Y, et al. Esophageal atresia: prognostic classification revisited. Surgery. 2009;145:675–81.
3. Malakounides G, Lyon P, Cross K, Pierro A, et al. esophageal atresia: improved outcome in high-risk groups revisited. Eur J Pediatr Surg. 2016;26(3):227–31.

CHAPTER 13

Gastrostomy without Laparotomy: A Percutaneous Endoscopic Technique

Michael WL Gauderer, Jeffrey L Ponsky, and Robert J Izant Jr.

Journal of Pediatric Surgery 1980; 15; 872–875.
Citations: *n* = 1,775 (!)

ABSTRACT

'A new technique has been developed to establish a tube feeding gastrostomy without a laparotomy. The procedure is particularly useful in high risk patients because general anesthesia is not usually required. The procedure is simple, safe, and rapid. It has been employed in 12 children (and 19 adults) with minimal morbidity and no mortality.'

COMMENTARY (MICHAEL GAUDERER)

It is interesting to note that, although the percutaneous endoscopic gastrostomy (PEG) had its origin in pediatric surgery, the astonishing success and spread was primarily due to its application to the adult population. At the time (1970s) I conceived the procedure, very few if any pediatric surgeons had access or were doing flexible endoscopy. In fact, the Children's Hospital of Philadelphia, where I had my fellowship, did not have a flexible endoscope. I initially considered rigid endoscopy – familiar to most pediatric surgeons at the time – but felt it was inadequate and possibly too risky. I also considered an imaging-guided procedure, but the radiologists at that time showed no interest. On the other hand, Dr Jeffrey Ponsky, whom I met after starting at University Hospitals in Cleveland, Ohio, had an early flexible scope of small enough caliber – as well as enthusiasm. Ironically, when I first presented the PEG at an APSA meeting, it was met with great curiosity but somewhat limited interest. The opposite occurred when it was presented to the gastroenterologists managing adult patients. It is worth noting that the PEG preceded laparoscopic surgery, the procedure generally preferred by pediatric surgeons, by several years. Although the original PEG report is the most quoted paper in the pediatric surgical literature, the skin-level device, or 'Button', that I also developed in Cleveland and published in the *Journal of Pediatric Surgery*, has received far less 'press' (1). As a colleague of mine commented: 'People think a gastrostomy Button has always existed'. It is interesting that the issue of gastrostomy, which is usually pretty straightforward in the pediatric population (feeding, decompression, medication), has

DOI: 10.1201/9781003341901-13

been the subject of much controversy in the adult population, particularly concerning the difficult end-of-life management.

COMMENTARY (JOE DAVIDSON)

Insertion of gastrostomy is one of the most commonly performed surgical procedures in children, and this is the most cited paper in the field. For some patients, it represents the only means of safe and secure enteral nutrition for their entire life, whereas for others it is a temporising measure through a period of need. The sheer frequency with which gastrostomy insertion is performed means that resource consumption and morbidity related to open surgery fast become a relevant issue. Various techniques, such as the Stamm gastrostomy (2), had been largely unchanged since the late nineteenth century, and it was not until 1971, more than 80 years later, that Michael Gauderer began to imagine an alternative procedure that might avoid much of the morbidity he was then encountering. However, the technique he envisaged required flexible endoscopy, something that was not present at his place of training; and so it was not until he joined the staff at Case Western Reserve University Hospital in Cleveland, Ohio, some years later and encountered Dr Jeffrey Ponsky, a paediatric surgeon and by then an already experienced endoscopist. Together they applied their principle to insert a gastrostomy tube using a 'railroad' (Figure 13.1) technique using only endoscopic visualisation of the stomach, calling this technique the percutaneous endoscopic gastrostomy (or PEG).

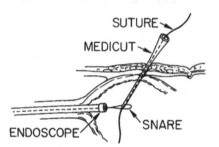

Figure 13.1 The thread, passed through the Medicut, is grasped with the snare of the endoscope. (Courtesy of Elsevier.)

This initial description of the PEG details outcomes from 12 children who had undergone the procedure. Note should be made that many of these children underwent the procedure under sedation or with only local anaesthesia. They report generally positive outcomes: all children had a successful placement of a gastrostomy tube. The complications presenting in the early introduction of the procedure are ones still encountered today: a tube needing upsizing, a tube migrating (prior to the introduction of an internal flange) and a 'buried bumper'. The authors also place a note of caution, that the relationship of the stomach and colon is such that when the stomach is inflated, although the colon is pushed inferiorly, the puncture should be made close to the costal margin to avoid a fistula.

In the 40-plus years (3) since the publication, there have been very few modifications to the technique of PEG insertion, with the exception of laparoscopic visualisation – which theoretically should eliminate the rare but reported incidence of gastrocolic fistula (4). A more recent alternative – the balloon gastrostomy – has the merits of not requiring anesthesia or endoscopy to change the device and is also the invention of Dr Gauderer (1). Many authors have proposed methods of primary insertion of balloon devices, although high-quality evidence to suggest a superiority in terms of complications and long-term outcomes is lacking (5).

REFERENCES

1. Gauderer MW, Picha GJ, Izant RJ Jr. The gastrostomy "button"–a simple, skin-level, nonrefluxing device for long-term enteral feedings. J Pediatr Surg. 1984;19(6):803–05.
2. Stamm M. Gastrostomy by a new method. Medical News. 1894;65, 324–26.
3. Gauderer MWL. Gastrointestinal feeding access - From idea to application. J Pediatr Surg. 2019;54:1099–1103.
4. Suksamanapun N, Mauritz F, Franken J, van der Zee D, van Herwaarden-Lindeboom M. Laparoscopic versus percutaneous endoscopic gastrostomy placement in children: Results of a systematic review and meta- analysis. J Minim Access Surg. 2017;13:81.
5. Davidson JR, Rae LD, Dhivyaa S, Wright H, Manasvia U, et al. Open primary button versus laparoscopic percutaneous endoscopic gastrostomy: results from a case-control study. J Pediatr Gastroenterol Nutr. 2021;72:e4–e9.

CHAPTER 14

Diamond-Shaped Anastomosis for Congenital Duodenal Obstruction

K Kimura, C Tsugawa, K Ogawa, Y Matsumoto, T Yamamoto, and S Asada

Archives of Surgery 1977; 112(10):1262–1263.
Citations: *n* = 67

ABSTRACT

This paper reports a new surgical technique to repair congenital duodenal obstruction in neonates. The conventional operation at the time being a side-to-side duodenojejunostomy.

Nine consecutive cases of duodenal obstruction (eight neonates and a four-year-old child who previously had a duodenojejunal anastomosis) underwent a 'diamond-shaped' side-to-side primary duodenoduodenostomy anastomosis.

After adequately mobilising the two ends of the duodenum, the 'diamond-shaped' joint started by making a transverse incision on the redundant side of the dilated proximal duodenal segment and a longitudinal incision on the antimesenteric border of the collapsed distal duodenal pouch (Figure 14.1). The anastomosis was fashioned by joining the apex of the incisions into the corresponding midpoints of the other duodenal side. This is started with two running sutures between the midpoint of the lower edge of the proximal segment and the proximal apex of the distal duodenum segment on either side. The anastomosis is then continued onto the anterior wall in a

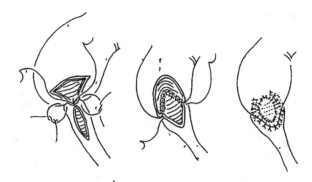

Figure 14.1 "Diamond" duodenojejunostomy.

DOI: 10.1201/9781003341901-14

similar fashion. In the original description a second layer of interrupted sutures is then placed to support the anastomosis.

Transanastomotic tubes (TAT) were not used intraoperatively, and none of the cases had a gastrostomy fashioned at the same time. Oral feeds were started from day three postoperatively and intravenous fluids were stopped by day six in five neonates.

There were two neonatal deaths related to sepsis and cerebral haemorrhage.

COMMENTARY (BASHAR ALDEIRI)

The 'Kimura' or 'Diamond' duodenoduodenostomy emerged at Kobe Children's Hospital in Japan, and the initial series took place between 1974 and 1977. Interestingly, it is not the initial series that is most cited for this new technique but rather the follow-on series that was published in 1990 reporting the outcomes of 44 cases treated at Kobe over 15 years using this technique ($n = 93$) (1). This report still had Kimura as a first author, despite that he himself had moved on to a new career at the University of Iowa in the USA.

This technique offered a better alternative to the surgical techniques practised, principally a side-to-side duodenojejunostomy, although a side to side duodenoduodenostomy was also emerging and commonly practised too (2, 3). The former was associated with a distal duodenum blind-loop and bile reflux gastritis, while the latter required extensive mobilisation of both duodenal pouches to allow for a tension-free anastomosis. It too was associated with poor duodenal drainage and often resulted in anastomotic stricture.

The novelty of the 'Kimura diamond' duodenoduodenostomy technique was in rearranging the axes of the two ends of the duodenum at time of anastomosis. This arrangement resulted in a wider duodenoduodenal anastomosis while averting the need for extensive mobilisation of the distal duodenal pouch (Figure 14.2).

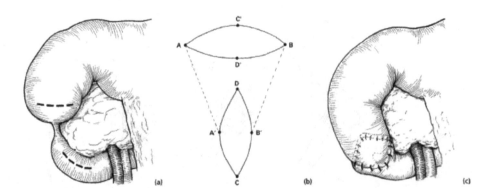

Figure 14.2 Kimura Diamond Duodenoduodenostomy.

The adoption of this new technique varied amongst the surgical community. Many embraced the new technique and reported better short-term outcomes (4), while others observed the new technique with some reservations. The proximity of the anastomosis to the biliary and pancreatic ducts was a particular source of concern potentially leading to kinking and biliary obstruction.

In the original description, Kimura et al. did not use a TAT or place a gastrostomy at the time of the repair. The general assumption at the time was that TATs were associated with higher incidence of anastomosis leaks, and hence their use was avoided. Despite this reservation, it is still common practice to leave a TAT (5). Infants with duodenal atresia tend to have poor gastric/duodenal emptying and have large gastric residuals for several days or even weeks postoperatively. Hence establishing gastric feeds early can be challenging.

Laparoscopic duodenal atresia repair has now been practised for about 20 years (6). Despite initial enthusiasm, the uptake of the laparoscopic approach has been relatively slow with a degree of scepticism amongst paediatric surgeons. A recent systematic review of eight large series did not show significant difference in complications rate, time to full enteral feeds or hospital stay between open and laparoscopic repair (7). Yet the data comparing the risk of anastomosis leak or stricture in the laparoscopic approach were based on three studies only. A recent analysis of a selected cohort of babies with duodenal atresia between 2016 and 2018 from a national North American database did not show difference in complications rate or time to full enteral nutrition between open and laparoscopic repairs (8). Interestingly, a laparoscopic repair was attempted in just over 10% of the infants in this cohort, and conversion to an open procedure was needed in almost a third. Laparoscopic duodenoduodenostomy is regarded as the most demanding paediatric laparoscopic procedure, and many have abandoned the technique.

Kimura's diamond duodenoduodenostomy remains the most widely practised technique in congenital duodenal obstruction to date.

REFERENCES

1. Kimura K, Mukohara N, Nishijima E, Muraji T, Tsugawa C, Matsumoto Y. Diamond-shaped anastomosis for duodenal atresia: an experience with 44 patients over 15 years. J Pediatr Surg. 1990;25:977–9.
2. Girvan DP, Stephens CA. Congenital intrinsic duodenal obstruction: a twenty-year review of its surgical management and consequences. J Pediatr Surg. 1974;9:833–9.
3. Wayne ER, Burrington JD. Management of 97 children with duodenal obstruction. Arch Surg. 1973;107:857–60.
4. Weber TR, Lewis JE, Mooney D, Connors R. Duodenal atresia: a comparison of techniques of repair. J Pediatr Surg. 1986;21:1133–6.
5. Biradar N, Gera P, Rao S. Trans-anastomotic tube feeding in the management of congenital duodenal obstruction: a systematic review and meta-analysis. Pediatr Surg Int. 2021;37:1489–98.

6. Bax NM, Ure BM, van der Zee DC, van Tuijl I. Laparoscopic duodenoduodenostomy for duodenal atresia. Surg Endosc. 2001;15(2):217.
7. Mentessidou A, Saxena AK. Laparoscopic repair of duodenal atresia: systematic review and meta-analysis. World J Surg. 2017;41:2178–84.
8. Weller JH, Engwall-Gill AJ, Westermann CR, et al. Laparoscopic versus open surgical repair of duodenal atresia: a NSQIP-pediatric analysis. J Surg Res. 2022;279:803–8.

CHAPTER 15

Intestinal Loop Lengthening – A Technique for Increasing Small Intestinal Length

Adrian Bianchi

Journal of Pediatric Surgery 1980; 15(2):145–151.
Citations: *n* = 405

ABSTRACT

This was a report of the development of a novel experimental technique in pigs. The procedure depended on an original insight into jejunal blood supply, whereby the mesenteric vessels diverged to either side of the intestine before entering its wall, leaving a dissectible mesenteric window (Figure 15.1). This allowed a longitudinal division of the bowel on both mesenteric and antimesenteric aspects, creating two lengths of viable bowel which could both then be tubularised. Functionally, this doubled available intestinal length while halving its diameter.

Seven pigs were studied with survival to at least 16 weeks in five of the seven animals. Some loops were just left as self-draining segments draining as an ostomy, while others were anastomosed together in an isoperistaltic fashion. Leakage led to the death of one animal. At the end of the experimental period, all loops were shown to be viable.

COMMENTARY (ADRIAN BIANCHI)

Longitudinal intestinal tailoring and lengthening (LILT) was conceived in 1977, when I was a registrar in paediatric surgery at Alder Hey Children's Hospital in Liverpool following consecutive laparotomies for antenatal short gut with its typical dilated proximal bowel, and for a long tubular small bowel duplication where a second patent fully vascularised bowel loop was situated along the antimesenteric border of the bowel. The realisation that the blood vessels entered the bowel wall one-third of the way up its lateral border, and the substantial safe avascular space within the mesentery beneath the bowel loop led to longitudinal division into two well-vascularised hemisegments that are tubularised and anastomosed end to end to create a functional full thickness isoperistaltic loop of half diameter and double length, and without loss of absorptive bowel. A research grant through Manchester Hospitals developed the concept in pigs, confirming lengthened loop viability, reliability and peristalsis, also exploring the adaptive response to a short bowel state.

DOI: 10.1201/9781003341901-15

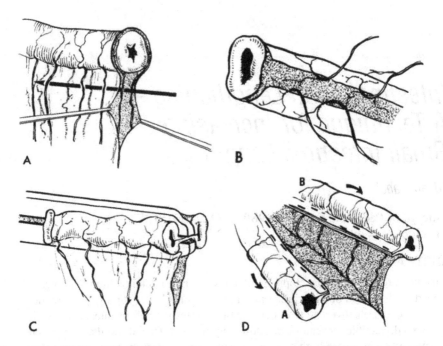

Figure 15.1 (A) Dissection between peritoneal leaves of mesentery. (B) Intervascular space. (C) Bowel loops between jaws of autostapler prior to division. (D) Hemiloops resulting from stapling and division of bowel. (Courtesy of Elsevier.)

LILT was presented at the 1979 Marseilles British Association of Paediatric Surgeons (BAPS) meeting, with Ovar Swenson as the chairman, and subsequently published (1). Initial derision was followed by increasing interest after Boeckman and Traylor from Akron, Ohio, reported the first clinical application to a four-year-old child in 1981 who successfully dispensed with intravenous feeding and resumed growth after LILT (2).

At the Royal Manchester Children's Hospital, and supported by Mr Ambrose Jolleys, I undertook our first clinical LILT in February 1982 for a six-week-old girl with short bowel following antenatal midgut loss. Postoperatively, despite intralipid-related severe liver dysfunction and within some three months, she established sufficient enteral absorption to dispense with parenteral nutrition. Her liver recovered and she grew through an uneventful childhood and adolescence to marriage and the birth of a son and a career in business. She died at 40 years of age from alcohol hepatotoxicity.

The crucial benefit from LILT is the reduction in the diameter of the dilated short bowel to propulsive proportions that eliminates the stasis, inflammation and sepsis associated with massive dilatation. The longer isopropulsive length prolongs contact time with healthy mucosa for increased absorption and enhanced mucosal adaptation. In addition to or replacing LILT, other surgical techniques such as serial transverse enteroplasty (STEP), spiral lengthening (SILT) and reversed antiperistaltic segments are now available. Adjuvant drug therapy (e.g. Clonidine, GLP-2) may enhance absorption and adaptation.

Current short bowel management is a long-term undertaking that has evolved to a holistic multidisciplinary autologous gastrointestinal rehabilitation plan (AGI-R) commencing with safe parenteral nutrition and 'bowel expansion' by a controllable intermittent obstruction to maximally dilate and elongate the residual bowel, thereby increasing the full thickness bowel wall for eventual bowel reconstruction. The intention is to allow the patient an enhanced family life and eventual nutrition on one's 'own bowel', avoiding bowel transplantation, which remains the final option.

COMMENTARY (MARK DAVENPORT)

Up until the 1980s, short bowel syndrome was widely regarded as an inevitably fatal condition. Although parenteral nutritional support was widely available, allowing survival beyond the neonatal period, the long-term prognosis, mainly due to the development of parenteral nutrition associated cholestasis and end-stage liver disease, was poor. Very few surgical manoeuvers were useful, though many had been tried, such as vagotomy and pyloroplasty, recirculating small bowel loops, loop reversal and preileal colon transposition. This novel procedure offered the potential of doubling available length and a way of improving peristaltic function, as most of the clinical causes of short bowel in infants (e.g., gastroschisis, intestinal atresia) resulted in residual intestinal dilatation, therefore impairing onward motility causing luminal content stagnation.

Adrian Bianchi, of Maltese extraction, settled in Manchester as a consultant paediatric surgeon during the 1980s. This together with a later paper published in a fairly low-impact journal in 1984 (1) was the basis for what became known as the 'Bianchi bowel-lengthening operation', though he always prefers the term 'longitudinal intestinal lengthening and tailoring'! Ironically, as he says in his preceding commentary, he wasn't the first to report the technique in a patient; that honour went to Boeckman and Traylor from Akron, Ohio, who operated on a four-year-old child in 1981 (2). Nonetheless, he slowly built up clinical experience in Manchester, attracting referrals and publishing his own series in 1999 (3). This paper describes 20 neonates and children who had undergone LILT. Long-term survival was achieved in 45%, with those survivors tending to have longer lengths of residual jejunum (> 40 cm) and had retained their ileocaecal values and by implication their colons. Indeed, there is very little experimental evidence in terms of absorption studies behind the technique and certainly none in the experimental animal models, but it does seem to work to increase tolerance of feeds without abdominal distension, allowing achievement of enteral autonomy in about 50%. Although the technique was originally described using a GIA™ stapler to aid the creation of the hemiloops, most surgeons hand-suture, and it can be a long, drawn-out operation because of it. Use of staples quickens the operating time, but the resulting hemiloops are fairly rigid. Perhaps surprisingly, leakage is not usually a problem, particularly if the loops are shown to be water-tight at the operating table. As to the timing of the surgery, in the early days the aim was to perform this as soon as practical and certainly before the onset of liver derangement. However, nowadays this stage is usually delayed. This is not only to try and select out those who will not adapt to conservative measures and definitely do need surgery, but also because, due to the advent of lipid-sparing parenteral nutrition regimens, liver injury is much less likely.

Currently, LILT is still in the repertoire of short bowel surgeons, though the STEP procedure (see Chapter 16) probably has more adherents for its ease of application and being relatively straightforward to do.

REFERENCES

1. Bianchi A. Intestinal lengthening: an experimental and clinical review. J R Soc Med. 1984;77(Suppl 3):35–41.
2. Boeckman CR, Traylor R. Bowel lengthening for short gut syndrome. J Pediatr Surg. 1981;16:996–99.
3. Bianchi A. Experience with longitudinal intestinal lengthening and tailoring. Eur J Pediatr Surg. 1999;9(4):256–59.

CHAPTER 16

Serial Transverse Enteroplasty (STEP): A Novel Bowel Lengthening Procedure

HB Kim, D Fauza, J Garza, J-T Oh, S Nurko, and T Jaksic

Journal of Pediatric Surgery 2003; 38: 425–429.
Citations: *n* = 316

ABSTRACT

This experimental study in pigs illustrated the use of a novel method of intestinal lengthening – serial transverse enteroplasty (STEP).

Young pigs (*n* = 6) underwent interposition of a reversed jejunal segment to produce proximal small bowel dilation. Five weeks later, the reversed segment was resected. Lengthening of the dilated bowel then was performed by serial transverse applications of a GIA™ stapler, from opposite directions, to create a zigzag channel (Figure 16.1).

Results: After bowel lengthening, all animals gained weight and showed no evidence of intestinal obstruction. Intraoperatively, immediately after STEP, the intestine was substantially elongated by about 68%. Six weeks after surgery, the lengthened intestinal segment became practically straight and, compared with the *in situ* control, remained significantly longer at about 64%. There was no difference in diameter between lengthened and the distal segments. There were no complications or deaths in the animals.

Conclusion: STEP significantly increases intestinal length without any evidence of obstruction. This procedure may be a safe and facile alternative for intestinal lengthening in children with short bowel syndrome

COMMENTARY (MARK DAVENPORT)

The STEP procedure was a product of animal and human studies in Boston, USA. Rather like the earlier Bianchi procedure, it was tested in pigs, but this time the authors deliberately produced jejunal dilatation in their model by reversing a jejunal segment. Fifteen to 20 firings of the GIA™ stapler were required in this study, and the authors orientated their staples lines to 90° and 270°. The authors suggest advantages over the aforementioned Bianchi procedure in that the technique is easier ('facile' in their abstract), has a much shorter anastomotic line (reducing the potential for leakage) and could even be done in cases where a Bianchi had been done but the bowel had redilated.

DOI: 10.1201/9781003341901-16

45

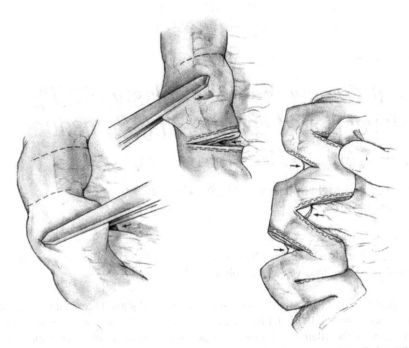

Figure 16.1   Schematic drawing of the serial transverse enteroplasty procedure. The small arrows show the direction of insertion of the GIA™ stapler and the sites of the mesenteric defects. The staplers are placed in the 90° and 270° orientations using the mesentery as the 0° reference point. (Courtesy of Elsevier.)

Unlike Bianchi, they did report later the same year the first clinical case of STEP in a two year old boy child with closing gastroschisis and initially a residual small intestinal length of 72 cm (1). He had already undergone a Bianchi operation to increase the length to 130 cm, but this didn't seem to be effective. Post-STEP follow-up is only reported to six months, but he apparently had improved enteral tolerance to about 50%.

There is some laboratory evidence of better functionality of the STEP procedure. In a Boston study (2) using the same pig model ($n = 10$) as before with induced proximal dilated jejunum by a reversed segment, 90% of the small bowel was resected, and in five pigs a STEP procedure was performed on the residual bowel. At six weeks, STEP pigs retained weight compared to a 17% loss in controls; they also had better D-xylose absorption and more normal triglyceride, albumin and vitamin D levels. Furthermore, bacterial overgrowth in the jejunum at sacrifice was present in 4/5 controls but no STEP animal.

An international registry was organized to popularise the technique, and collected data from 50 hospitals in 13 countries during the period 2004–2010, reporting in 2013 (3). In this, 111 patients were registered, but only 97 had sufficient data for analysis.

Of these, 11 died and five subsequently underwent intestinal transplantation. In a subset of 78 infants > 7 days old, enteral autonomy was achieved in 37 (47%) at a median of 21 months. As with the earlier Bianchi operation, and very predictably, the best results occurred in those with the longest residual intestine pre-STEP and those who had no evidence of liver disease.

There has been a recent systematic analysis (4) on 308 reported cases from 23 reports in both adults and children. Overall, in the pediatric subgroup ($n = 180$) with gastroschisis and intestinal atresia as the two principle pathologies, 32% achieved enteral autonomy, with a mortality rate of 5%.

REFERENCES

1. Kim HB, Lee PW, Garza J, et al. Serial transverse enteroplasty for short bowel syndrome: a case report. J Pediatr Surg. 2003;38:881–885.
2. Chang RW, Javid PJ, Oh J-T, et al. Serial Transverse Enteroplasty enhances intestinal function in a model of short bowel syndrome. Ann Surg. 2006;243:223–228.
3. Jones BA, Hull MA, Potanos KM, et al. Report of 111 consecutive patients enrolled in the International Serial Transverse Enteroplasty (STEP) Data Registry: a retrospective observational study. J Am Coll Surg. 2013;216(3):438–46. doi: 10.1016/j.jamcollsurg.2012.12.018
4. Lauro A, Santoro A, Cirocchi R, et al. Serial transverse enteroplasty (STEP) in case of short bowel syndrome: did we achieve our goal? A systematic review. Updates Surg. 2022;74(4):1209–1223. doi: 10.1007/s13304-022-01316-3

CHAPTER 17

Neonatal Necrotizing Enterocolitis. Therapeutic Decisions Based upon Clinical Staging

MJ Bell, JL Ternberg, RD Feigin, JP Keating, R Marshall, L Barton, and T Brotherton

Annals of Surgery 1978; 187(1):1–7
Citations: n = 2,497!!

ABSTRACT

'A method of clinical staging for infants with necrotizing enterocolitis (NEC) is proposed (Table 17.1). On the basis of assigned stage at the time of diagnosis, 48 infants were treated with graded intervention. For Stage I infants, vigorous diagnostic and supportive measures are appropriate. Stage II infants are treated medically, including parenteral and gavage aminoglycoside antibiotic, and Stage III patients require operation. All Stage I patients survived, and 32 of 38 Stage II and III

Table 17.1 NEC Staging System Based upon Historical, Clinical and Radiographic Data

STAGE I (Suspect)

a. Any one or more historical factors producing perinatal stress.
b. Systemic manifestations – temperature instability, lethargy, apnea, bradycardia.
c. Gastrointestinal manifestations: poor feeding, increasing pregavage residuals, emesis (may be bilious or test positive for occult blood), mild abdominal distension. Occult blood may be present in stool (no fissure).
d. Abdominal radiographs show distension with mild ileus.

STAGE II (Definite)

a. Any one or more historical factors.
b. Above signs and symptoms plus persistent occult or gross gastrointestinal bleeding; marked abdominal distension.
c. Abdominal radiographs show significant intestinal distension with ileus; small bowel separation (edema in bowel wall or peritoneal fluid), unchanging or persistent 'rigid' bowel loops, pneumatosis intestinalis, portal vein gas.

STAGE III (Advanced)

a. Any one or more historical factors.
b. Above signs and symptoms plus deterioration of vital signs, evidence of septic shock or marked gastrointestinal hemorrhage.
c. Abdominal radiographs may show pneumoperitoneum in addition to others listed in Stage II c.

Bell MJ, Ternberg JL, Feigin RD, Keating JP, Marshall R, Barton L, Brotherton T. *Annals of Surgery* 1978; 187(1):1–7

DOI: 10.1201/9781003341901-17

patients (85%) survived the acute episode of NEC. Bacteriologic evaluation of the gastrointestinal microflora in these neonates has revealed a wide range of enteric organisms, including anaerobes. Enteric organisms were cultured from the blood of four infants dying of NEC. Sequential cultures of enteric organisms reveal an alteration of flora during gavage antibiotic therapy. These studies support the use of combination antimicrobial therapy in the treatment of infants with NEC.'

COMMENTARY (JOE DAVIDSON)

This paper by Dr Martin Bell and colleagues from St Louis Children's Hospital, published in *Annals of Surgery* in 1978, came at a time when the features of NEC and risk factors had been largely well documented. However, consistent definitions were fundamentally lacking – leading to great variance in treatment strategies and outcomes (1). Many contributing factors have since been described with significant scientific rigour, with randomized trials performed related to enteral feeding practices (2), along with detailed scientific study of the intestinal microbiome (3) and inflammatory cascade (4) as they relate to disease onset and progression.

Bell's staging system was conceived in order to guide a clinical treatment protocol for neonates with a diagnosis of NEC (see Table 17.1). The features of Stage I NEC require considerable scrutiny to exclude other conditions, indeed many clinicians opt not to report cases of Stage I NEC owing to considerable diagnostic uncertainty and variability between centres (5). The staging was modified by Walsh and Kliegman to divide each stage into two, differentiating on additional symptoms such as fresh rectal bleeding (IA/IB) and presence of pneumoperitoneum (IIIA/IIIB) (6).

It is important to bear in mind that Bell's staging was never intended to be used as diagnostic criteria for NEC. Rather, it was intended to guide treatment for newborns suspected of the condition on clinical grounds – within which risk factors such as prematurity might already be factored in. This is a relevant distinction, as many of the aspects of the criteria (such as abdominal distension, bilious aspirates or feed intolerance) have extremely low specificity. Furthermore, a lack of filtering of cases of spontaneous intestinal perforation additionally contaminates data in studies that report using this system as a means of case definition – at the time of Bell's initial description, use of indomethacin and prevalence of extreme prematurity would have been considerably lower than today, hence the authors might be forgiven for this. Further scrutiny of Bell's staging has also referred to other confounding diagnoses that may confuse matters that may be more common in the neonatal unit of today, including viral enteritis and cow's milk protein allergy as well as underlining distinct features of NEC, where it may be caused by local ischaemia or in cases associated with congenital cardiac disease (7).

Bell's staging (or its modification) has synchronised almost completely with clinical studies reporting NEC outcomes for more than four decades (8). Identification of high-risk infants for prophylactic measures, early identification and stratification of disease and consistent definitions within and between surgical centres are truly essential to continue to drive progress forward in this challenging condition.

REFERENCES

1. Obladen M. Necrotizing enterocolitis – 150 years of fruitless search for the cause. Neonatology. 2009;96:203–210.
2. Berseth CL, Bisquera JA, & Paje VU. Prolonging small feeding volumes early in life decreases the incidence of necrotizing enterocolitis in very low birth weight infants. Pediatrics. 2003;111:529–534.
3. Warner BB, Deych E, et al. Gut bacteria dysbiosis and necrotising enterocolitis in very low birthweight infants: a prospective case-control study. Lancet. 2016;387:1928–1936.
4. Kovler ML, Gonzalez Salazar AJ, et al. Toll-like receptor 4-mediated enteric glia loss is critical for the development of necrotizing enterocolitis. Sci Transl Med. 2021;13(612):eabg3459. doi: 10.1126/scitranslmed.abg3459.
5. Patel RM, Ferguson J, McElroy SJ, Khashu M, & Caplan MS. Defining necrotizing enterocolitis: current difficulties and future opportunities. Pediatr Res. 2020;88:10–15.
6. Walsh MC & Kliegman RM. Necrotizing enterocolitis: treatment based on staging criteria. Pediatr Clin North Am. 1986;33:179–201.
7. Gordon PV, Swanson JR, Attridge JT, & Clark R. Emerging trends in acquired neonatal intestinal disease: is it time to abandon Bell's criteria? J Perinatol. 2007;27:661–671.
8. Battersby C, Santhalingam T, Costeloe K, & Modi N. Incidence of neonatal necrotising enterocolitis in high-income countries: a systematic review. Arch Dis Child Fetal Neonatal Ed. 2018;103:F182–F189.

CHAPTER 18

Laparotomy versus Peritoneal Drainage for Necrotizing Enterocolitis and Perforation

R Lawrence Moss, RA Dimmitt, DC Barnhart, (…), D Zelterman, and BL Silverman

New England Journal of Medicine 2006; 354:2225–2234
Citations *n* = 292

ABSTRACT

Perforated necrotising enterocolitis (NEC) is a major cause of morbidity and mortality in premature infants, and the optimal treatment is uncertain. This multicentre randomized trial was designed to compare outcomes of primary peritoneal drainage with laparotomy and bowel resection in preterm infants with perforated necrotising enterocolitis.

Methods: Randomization of 117 preterm infants (<34 weeks of gestation) with birth weights <1,500 g and perforated necrotizing enterocolitis at 15 pediatric centres to undergo primary peritoneal drainage (PPD) or laparotomy with bowel resection (LAP). Postoperative care was standardized. The primary outcome was survival at 90 days postoperatively. Secondary outcomes included dependence on parenteral nutrition 90 days postoperatively and length of hospital stay.

Results: There was no difference in the mortality (PPD, 19/55 [34%] vs LAP, 62/62 [35%]; P = 0.92) at 90 days postoperatively There was no difference in dependence on total parenteral nutrition (PPD, 17/36 [47%] vs LAP, 16/40 [40%]; P = 0.53). The mean (±SD) length of hospitalisation for the 76 infants who were alive 90 days after operation was also similar (PPD, 126 ± 58 days vs LAP, 116 ± 56 days, P = 0.43). Subgroup analyses stratified according to the presence or absence of radiographic evidence of extensive necrotizing enterocolitis (pneumatosis intestinalis), gestational age of < 25 weeks, and serum pH < 7.30 at presentation showed no significant advantage of either treatment in any group.

Five infants (one death) in the PPD underwent salvage early laparotomy and 16 delayed (> 26 days) laparotomy for stricture etc. (two deaths).

Conclusions: The type of operation performed for perforated necrotising enterocolitis does not influence survival or other clinically important early outcomes in preterm infants.

DOI: 10.1201/9781003341901-18

COMMENTARY (JOE DAVIDSON)

Paediatric surgical trials, and especially those about neonatal surgery, are notoriously difficult to design, recruit and complete. NEC is still one of the leading causes of morbidity and mortality amongst premature infants and the most common reason for mortality in paediatric surgery. Larry Moss and colleagues across 15 neonatal centres in the United States conducted the first RCT for the initial surgical management of NEC. The concept of primary peritoneal drainage had previously been identified, many years before, as a temporising or even curative measure for premature infants with intestinal perforation and is associated with the work of Sigmund Ein in Toronto (1). However, many infants still required laparotomy, and the role of only draining in perforated NEC was controversial.

Where the study left questions unanswered was in its ability to statistically evaluate differences between subgroups. Alan Flake, in his *New England Journal of Medicine* (NEJM) editorial accompanying the article, rightly refers to the fact that there were insufficient numbers to detect outcome differences between the smallest infants (i.e. <1,000 g, for whom peritoneal drainage might have been considered the sensible alternative) (2).

Since the publication of this trial, two further studies have also been published. Clair Rees and colleagues from Great Ormond Street, London, led an international randomized trial (NET) comparing the same two treatment options (3). The study ($n = 69$) ultimately closed before reaching its recruitment target, but similarly showed little difference in mortality between the two treatment options. However, salvage laparotomy was much more frequently used to achieve this, and PPD was effective as a definitive treatment in only 4/35 (11%) surviving infants. The infants included were smaller (≤1,000 g vs ≤1,500 g), and focal intestinal perforation was included along with NEC (as it had been in the Moss study). A further analysis of this dataset (4) also failed to show improvements in the pathophysiological measurements of sick infants in the PPD group.

More recently, Martin Blakely et al. published a much larger ($n = 310$) American multicenter study with outcomes of death or neurodevelopmental impairment at 22–24 (corrected age) months (5). Similar to both previous studies, this study identified no essential difference in the outcome overall but did recognise a clear effect of treatment based on previous diagnosis. Blakely et al. also pioneered a fresh approach to statistical evaluation using Bayesian analysis as opposed to trying to reach a preset P value of 0.05 for adjudication. Thus, they identified that a diagnosis of NEC had a 97% posterior probability of treatment benefit of laparotomy compared to only 18% in cases of focal intestinal perforation. This would reinforce the beliefs of many surgeons – that the necrotic process in NEC needs to be resected – and makes a clear case for the need to discriminate accurately between the two conditions.

REFERENCES

1. Ein SH, Marshall DG, Girvan D. Peritoneal drainage under local anesthesia for perforations from necrotizing enterocolitis. J Pediatr Surg. 1977;12:963–967.
2. Flake AW. Necrotizing enterocolitis in preterm infants—is laparotomy necessary? N Engl J Med. 2006;354:2275–2276.
3. Rees CM, Eaton S, Kiely EM, et al. peritoneal drainage or laparotomy for neonatal bowel perforation? A randomized controlled trial. Ann Surg. 2008;248:44–51.
4. Rees CM, Eaton S, Khoo AK, Kiely EM, Pierro A. Peritoneal drainage does not stabilize extremely low birth weight infants with perforated bowel: data from the NET Trial. J Pediatr Surg. 2010;45:324–329.
5. Blakely ML, Tyson JE, Lally KP, et al. Initial laparotomy versus peritoneal drainage in extremely low birthweight infants with surgical necrotizing enterocolitis or isolated intestinal perforation: a multicenter randomized clinical trial. Ann Surg. 2021;274:e370–e380. doi: 10.1097/SLA.0000000000005099

CHAPTER 19

Pediatric Appendicitis Score

Madan Samuel

Journal of Pediatric Surgery 2002; 37(6):877–881.
Citations: $n = 351$

ABSTRACT

Aim: Morbidity in children treated with appendicitis results either from late diagnosis or negative appendicectomy. A prospective analysis of the efficacy of a Pediatric Appendicitis Score (PAS) for early diagnosis of appendicitis.

Methods: One thousand one hundred and seventy children (aged four to 15 years) with abdominal pain suggestive of acute appendicitis were evaluated prospectively (in the last five years). Group 1 ($n = 734$) consisted of patients with appendicitis, and group 2 ($n = 436$) nonappendicitis. Multiple linear logistic regression analysis of all clinical and investigative variables was performed for a model comprising eight variables to form a diagnostic score.

Results: A total of 770 children underwent surgical exploration, and of these 36 (4.8%) did not have appendicitis. In the nonappendicitis group, 400/436 did not undergo surgery and were treated conservatively. All eight variables were significantly different ($P < 0.001$). These variables in order of their diagnostic index were (1) cough/percussion/hopping tenderness in the right-lower quadrant of the abdomen (0.96), (2) anorexia (0.88), (3) pyrexia (0.87), (4) nausea/emesis (0.86), (5) tenderness over the right iliac fossa (0.84), (6) leukocytosis (0.81), (7) polymorphonuclear neutrophilia (0.80) and (8) migration of pain (0.80). Each of these variables was assigned a score of 1, except for physical signs (1 and 5), which were scored 2 to obtain a total of 10.

The Pediatric Appendicitis Score had a sensitivity of 1, specificity of 0.92, positive predictive value of 0.96 and negative predictive value of 0.99.

Conclusion: Pediatric appendicitis score is a simple, relatively accurate diagnostic tool for accessing an acute abdomen and diagnosing appendicitis in children.

COMMENTARY (BASHAR ALDEIRI)

This study was conducted in an era were negative appendicectomy rates were reported to be as high as 30% of cases. The current study was obviously inspired by Alfredo Alvarado's (1), which was published in 1986 based on a retrospective cohort of

DOI: 10.1201/9781003341901-19

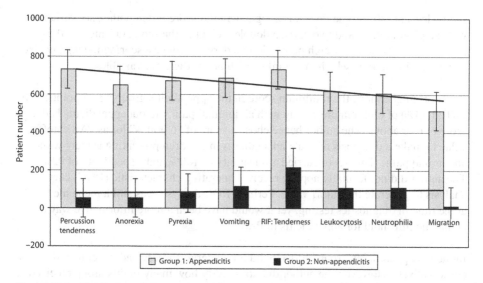

Figure 19.1 Distribution of diagnostic variables between Group 1(appendicitis) and Group 2 (nonappendicitis).

305 patients of mixed adults and children seen at the Nazareth Hospital, Philadelphia. Compared to that work, this was prospective, four times larger and paediatric only. Indeed, seven of eight variables suggested by Alvarado were present in the PAS. While in theory rebound tenderness was excluded from PAS, as it was regarded as a cruel test to subject a child to (Figure 19.1).

The study was conducted at St George's Hospital in South London and Southampton General Hospital in Southeast England. The only exclusion criterion was children with an established appendix mass, presumably confirmed at time of surgery. The author analysed 13 variables: patient age, gender, anorexia, nausea/vomiting, migration of pain from umbilical area to right iliac fossa (RIF), RIF tenderness on palpation, RIF tenderness on hopping/coughing/percussion, pyrexia, total white blood cell count, differential white blood cell count, urinalysis and as the thing to be predicted – histology of the appendix.

Each variables' sensitivity and specificity were calculated based on histological confirmation of acute appendicitis in children who underwent surgery or establishing an alternative medical diagnosis to appendicitis in those who did not. Subsequently, each variable was assigned a diagnostic index (weight), which was the sum of the true positive and true negative cases for a diagnosis of acute appendicitis. These markers were then further tested in a linear regression model to determine their individual diagnostic weight overall and in relation to each other. A PAS score comprised the best eight variables with the best correlation. Percussion tenderness (including when exacerbated with coughing or hopping) yielded the highest diagnostic weight (96%), and migration of abdominal pain from the periumbilical area to the right iliac fossa scored least at (80%). The PAS was assigned a total score of ten points; six variables were single-weighted and two carried double-weight in the score. Of interest, the author elected to double-weigh percussion tenderness (highest scoring index), but also tenderness in the RIF, which only ranked fifth out of the eight variables.

In the original cohort, the minimum score in the appendicitis group was 6 points: only 37/1170 (3%) of children presenting with abdominal pain without appendicitis had a score of 6 or above. The author hence chose a score of "6 points" for as PAS cutoff value to make a diagnosis of acute appendicitis in children presenting acutely with abdominal pain. This score carried a sensitivity of 100% and a specificity of 92%. The author did not formally apply a receiver operating characteristic (ROC) curve analysis to generate the cutoff value. Perhaps ROC analysis was still a niche method at the time in diagnostics testing, yet it would have been a more informative way to define the threshold for appendicitis in PAS.

In the nonappendicitis group, 400/436 did not undergo surgery and were treated conservatively. However, the author did not specify how many in this group received antibiotics before a final diagnosis was made. There may well have been a cohort in this group who have, nonintentionally, received a nonoperative treatment of acute appendicitis, and how this has affected the validity of the score is a question that will never find an answer.

In an addendum to the original publication, the author assessed the validity of the PAS in a separate prospective cohort of 66 children presenting with abdominal pain. The PAS demonstrated much less impressive statistics – a sensitivity of 1, specificity of 0.87, positive predictive value of 0.90 and a negative predictive value of 1 using a cutoff of ≤ 5 for nonappendicitis and ≥ 8 for appendicitis.

More than two decades have passed since the publication of the first paediatric appendicitis score, yet the subject is still of interest to many clinicians and researchers. There are over a dozen appendicitis scores that have been proposed for children, and there are over 90 publications to date validating and comparing their use (2).

REFERENCES

1. Alvarado A. A practical score for the early diagnosis of acute appendicitis. Ann Emerg Med. 1986;15(5):557–564. doi: 10.1016/s0196-0644(86)80993-3. PMID: 3963537. (Citations 306).
2. RIFT Study Group on behalf of the West Midlands Research Collaborative. Appendicitis risk prediction models in children presenting with right iliac fossa pain (RIFT study): a prospective, multicentre validation study. Lancet Child Adolesc Health. 2020;4(4):271–280.

CHAPTER 20

A Rectal Suction Biopsy Tube for Use in the Diagnosis of Hirschsprung's Disease

Helen Rae Noblett

Journal of Pediatric Surgery 1969; 4(4):406–409.
Citations: *n* = 98

Experience with Rectal Suction Biopsy in the Diagnosis of Hirschsprung's Disease

Peter E Campbell and Helen Rae Noblett

Journal of Pediatric Surgery 1969; 4:410–415.
Citations: *n* = 64

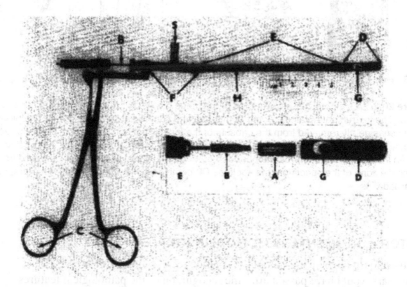

Figure 20.1 Rectal suction biopsy tube assembled for use. Inset: biopsy capsule and cylindrical knife dismantled; (A) cylindrical knife; (B) central operating wire; (C) Jackson-Negus handle; (D) biopsy capsule; (E) flexible tube; (F) suction handle unit; (G) side aperture; (H) longitudinal marker; (S) side arm for connection to suction.

DOI: 10.1201/9781003341901-20

ABSTRACT

These two papers were published in the same issue of the *Journal of Pediatric Surgery*. The first simply described the new device (Figure 20.1) with the second one describing actual results in 85 patients. Excluding 14 patients for whom the biopsy material was unsatisfactory due to causes subsequently corrected in the second half of the series, all of the remaining 71 patients were diagnosed correctly in reference to Hirschsprung's disease. The biopsy specimen should be taken above the hypoganglionic zone, 3 cm cranial of the pectinate line, with absence of ganglion cells from a serially sectioned suction biopsy specimen yielding at least 2 mm² of submucosa being diagnostic of Hirschsprung's disease (Figure 20.2).

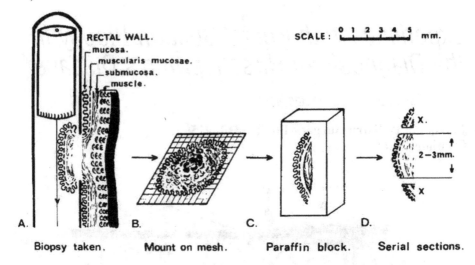

Figure 20.2 A schematic representation of the steps involved in taking a mucosal suction biopsy. The instrument obtains a dome of mucosa and superficial submucosa (A). The biopsy specimen is gently removed from the capsule of the instrument and laid flat on Teflon gauze, mucosal surface uppermost (B). After fixation in neutral formalin, the specimen is processed to paraffin in the routine manner and embedded on edge (C). Serial sections are prepared from the middle zone of the specimen, the sections (X) coming from the first and last quarters, being discarded (D).

EDITOR's COMMENTARY (JOE DAVIDSON)

It is hard to imagine an era before the cot-side rectal biopsy. However, 20 or more years would have passed after the recognition of the pathological features of Hirschsprung's disease before the use of suction biopsy of the rectum became commonplace. Helen Noblett, an Australian junior paediatric surgeon at the time, and a pathologist colleague, Peter Campbell from the Royal Children's Hospital, Melbourne, published their experience with a device of their own creation in 1969.

The concept of suction biopsy of the rectal submucosa was not new. In fact, William O Dobbins III and Alexander H Bill Jr from the University of Washington had published prominently in the *New England Journal of Medicine* their experiences with suction biopsy in a selection of 149 patients with varying pathologies and showing that ganglion cells could normally be seen (1). Nevertheless, it was Noblett (1933–2020), with a forceps that would bear her name (rather than Campbell's) into the next millennium, who described the particular relevance and utilisation of this in the diagnosis and workup of children with Hirschsprung's disease.

The use of suction biopsy in Hirschsprung's was not immediately popular because of the preference of pathologists to examine for the presence of ganglion cells in Auerbach's plexus between the longitudinal and circular muscle layers of the colon (2). However, it was recognised that the limits of aganglionosis in the submucosal Meissner's plexus closely matched those of Auerbach's, leading to a slow movement towards the less precarious sampling of this layer only during sigmoidoscopy.

Noblett's forceps allowed for biopsies to be taken from the rectal mucosa in an awake patient; they presented a series of 85 patients with and without Hirschsprung's in whom no complications of the procedure were reported but an inadequate biopsy rate of 37% (19/52) in their initial experience (falling to 0%, 0/116) once modifications to their technique and their instrument had been made). Inadequate biopsy remains a constant headache for the paediatric surgical junior (4), and Noblett discusses a few factors that may affect this in her experience with the device. First, she notes that the use of enemas may result in oedema of the mucosal layer, resulting in a biopsy that insufficiently samples the underlying submucosa. Second, digital examination of the rectal passage may lead to inflammatory changes that make the histological analysis more challenging. Finally, a clear description of the ideal biopsy is made:

> The mucosa appeared as a small shiny dome of tan tissue while the submucosa on the reverse aspect was a button of grey tissue, readily distinguished from the overlying tan mucosa. A submucosal lymphoid follicle, when present, also appeared yellow-tan and contrasted with the grey of the nonlymphoid submucosa. When the deep surface of a specimen appeared tan another biopsy was obtained immediately, as specimens containing lymphoid tissue usually proved unsatisfactory for diagnosis.

Perhaps recognition of the ideal use of the instrument as described by its creator may save us some headaches still!

REFERENCES

1. Dobbins WO, Bill AH. Diagnosis of Hirschsprung's disease excluded by rectal suction biopsy. New Eng J Med. 1965;272:990–3.

2. Swenson O, Fisher J, MacMahon H. Rectal biopsy as an aid in the diagnosis of Hirschsprung's disease. N Engl J Med. 1955;253:632–5.
3. Gherardi G. Pathology of the ganglionic-aganglionic junction in congenital megacolon. Arch Pathol. 1960;69:520–3.
4. Hall NJ, Kufeji D, Keshtgar A. Out with the old and in with the new: a comparison of rectal suction biopsies with traditional and modern biopsy forceps. J Pediatr Surg. 2009;44:395–8.

CHAPTER 21

Point Mutations Affecting the Tyrosine Kinase Domain of the RET Proto-Oncogene in Hirschsprung's Disease

Romeo G, Ronchetto P, Luo Y, Barone V, et al. Point mutations affecting the tyrosine kinase domain of the RET proto-oncogene in Hirschsprung's disease

Nature 1994; 367, 377–378.
Citations: *n* = 651

Mutations of the RET Proto-Oncogene in Hirschsprung's Disease

Edery P, Lyonnet S, Mulligan L. et al.

Nature 1994; 367, 378–380.
Citations *n* = 641

ABSTRACT (COMBINED AND EDITED)

Hirschsprung's disease (HD) is a genetic disorder of neural crest development affecting one in 5,000 births. It is characterised by the absence of intramural ganglion cells in the hindgut, which often results in partial to complete intestinal obstruction during the first years of life. Segregation analyses have suggested incompletely penetrant dominant inheritance in familial HSCR. Recently, a gene for HSCR was mapped to chromosome 10q11.2. No recombination was observed between the disease locus and the locus for the RET proto-oncogene, a protein tyrosine kinase gene expressed in the cells derived from the neural crest. Here we report nonsense and missense mutations in the extracellular domain of RET protein (exons 2, 3, 5 and 6). Mutations in the extracellular cysteine-rich domain of RET have been identified previously in patients with multiple endocrine neoplasia (MEN) type 2A, and a targeted mutation in the tyrosine kinase domain of the same gene produces intestinal aganglionosis and kidney agenesis in homozygous transgenic mice. Thus, germ-line mutations of the RET

DOI: 10.1201/9781003341901-21

gene may contribute either to developmental anomalies in HSCR or to inherited predisposition to cancer in MEN 2A. Our results support the hypothesis that RET, in addition to its potential role in tumorigenesis, plays a critical role in the embryogenesis of the mammalian enteric nervous system.

Point mutations affecting the tyrosine kinase domain of the *RET* proto-oncogene in Hirschsprung's disease

Giovanni Romeo, Patrizia Ronchetto, Yin Luo, Virginia Barone, Marco Seri, Isabella Ceccherini, Barbara Pasini, Renata Bocciardi, Margherita Lerone, Helena Kääriäinen* & Giuseppe Martucciello

Istituto Giannina Gaslini, 16148 Genova-Quarto, Italy
* Department of Medical Genetics, University of Helsinki,
Helsinki SF 00014, Finland

Mutations of the *RET* proto-oncogene in Hirschsprung's disease

Patrick Edery*, Stanislas Lyonnet*, Lois M. Mulligan†, Anna Pelet*, Eleanore Dow‡, Laurent Abel§, Susan Holder‖, Claire Nihoul-Fékété*, Bruce A. J. Ponder† & Arnold Munnich*¶

* Service de Génétique Médicale, Clinique Chirurgicale Infantile et Unité de Recherches sur les Handicaps Génétiques de l'Enfant, INSERM U-393, Hôpital Necker-Enfants Malades, 149, rue de Sèvres, 75743 Paris cedex 15, France
† CRC Human Cancer Genetics Research Group, Department of Pathology, University of Cambridge, Tennis Court Road, Cambridge CB2 1QP, UK
‡ Department of Biochemistry and Molecular Genetics, St Mary's Hospital Medical School, London W2 1PG, UK
§ Unité INSERM U-194, Hôpital de la Pitié-Salpétrière, 75634 Paris cedex 13, France
‖ Mothercare Unit of Clinical Genetics, Institute of Child Health, Guilford Street, London WC1N 1EH, UK

COMMENTARY (JOE DAVIDSON)

Bodian and Carter at Great Ormond Street Hospital (1), London, and Passarge in Cincinnati, Ohio (2), began to describe the inheritance patterns of HD in larger numbers of affected families. These studies showed a clearly increased incidence in males and children with trisomy 21, but far too few affected relatives for a monogenic recessive condition.

In 1994, the journal *Nature* published back-to-back letters from the research teams of Kaarlainen (Helsinki, Finland) and Martuciello (Genoa, Italy) together with Arnold Munnich (Paris, France), detailing their respective, independent observations of mutations in the RET proto-oncogene in Hirschsprung's patients. Both studies were based upon observations made by a collaborative effort between the two groups published in *Nature Genetics* the previous year (3); that a patient with total colonic aganglionosis had a partial deletion in the long-arm of chromosome 10 (10q11.2–q21.2), which was mapped against 15 other Hirschsprung's affected families to suggest a dominant gene for HD to be within this region (also associated with other neurocristopathies).

Both published studies utilised single-strand conformation polymorphism (SSCP), a relatively new technique designed to examine for small-scale sequence variations and point mutations using electrophoretic properties of amplified DNA from the patient samples. Both teams explored exons from the RET gene, in unrelated patients and in known familial cases, identifying prevalent mutations in specific coding regions of the gene that seemed to be associated with Hirschsprung's cases; however, these were generally in distinct sites to those regions that have been typically mutated in cases of multiple endocrine neoplasia type 2 (MEN2A and MEN2B are cancer syndromes known to be related to mutations in the RET gene). An interesting point to note is that silent mutations in the gene were noted in relatives of affected individuals, strengthening the theory of complex inheritance.

Edery et al. conclude that the mutations leading to Hirschsprung's were likely inactivating or abrogating the gene product, whereas those leading to MEN were activating mutations of the proto-oncogene. However, subsequent to this study, there have since been patients identified in whom both MEN syndrome and HD coexist, suggesting both activating and inactivating mutations in the same gene and seemingly focussing on a specific mutation in an extracellular cysteine-rich domain of exon 10. With rapid advances in sequencing technology, many genetic associations have now been recognised to exist with HD. Yet the RET gene remains by far the most significant – comprising 50% of familial cases and present in 15–20% of sporadic cases. As such, these early studies must be considered highly important for the risk counselling of patients and their families.

REFERENCES

1. Bodian M, Carter CO, Ward BC. Hirschsprung's disease. Lancet. 1951;1(6650):302–9. doi: 10.1016/s0140-6736(51)92290-8.

2. Passarge E. The genetics of Hirschsprung's disease. Evidence for heterogeneous etiology and a study of sixty-three families. N Engl J Med. 1967;276(3):138–43. doi: 10.1056/ NEJM196701192760303. PMID: 4224912.
3. Lyonnet S, Bolino A, Pelet A, Abel L, et al. A gene for Hirschsprung disease maps to the proximal long arm of chromosome 10. Nat Genet. 1993;4(4):346–50. doi: 10.1038/ ng0893-346. PMID: 8401580.

CHAPTER 22

Endorectal "Pull-Through" without Preliminary Colostomy in Neonates with Hirschsprung's Disease

So HB, Schwartz DL, Becker JM, Daum F, and Schneider KM

Journal of Pediatric surgery 1980; 15:470–471
Citations: $n = 148$

ABSTRACT

The diagnosis of Hirschsprung's disease in the newborn does not mandate the performance of a preliminary colostomy. Enterocolitis can be adequately and safely treated by a precise regimen of colonic irrigations. The endorectal "pull-through" (PT) procedure is safe and effective when performed in the neonatal period. Long-term follow-up is necessary to evaluate possible late complications.

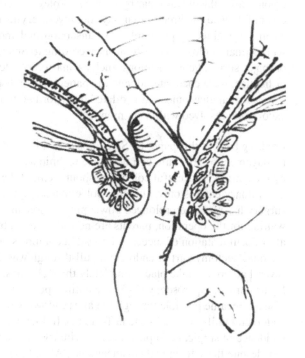

KEY POINTS

- Ten-year series of 20 patients treated with neonatal endorectal pull-through (abdominal).
- Preferential repeated colonic irrigation after birth with neonatal pull-through (before 30 days).
- First description of neonatal PT in Hirschsprung's disease (HD) without colostomy

DOI: 10.1201/9781003341901-22

EXPERT COMMENTARY (MIKKO PAKARINEN)

One-stage pull-through surgery for Hirschsprung's disease (HD) started to gain popularity among pediatric surgeons during the last two decades of the twentieth century. Prior to that, the functional intestinal obstruction had been initially dealt with by performing preliminary enterostomy, which also effectively prevented enterocolitis while postponing the pull-through beyond the neonatal period.

In 1980, Henry So, together with a group of pediatric surgeons from New York, described 20 neonates who underwent primary endorectal pull-through. The results were initially presented at the Surgical Section of the American Academy of Pediatrics (AAP) in 1979 and published in the *Journal of Pediatric Surgery* the following year.

Bowel preparation for the surgery included one to two days saline irrigation of the colon until effluent was clear by passing a Foley catheter all the way to the right colon, followed by three to four days neomycin-erythromycin bowel preparation. Their surgical technique combined transabdominal and transanal mucosectomy with primary colo-anal anastomosis according to Soave and Boley (1, 2). No deaths or major surgical complications, such as anastomotic leakage, strictures, abscesses or fistulae, were encountered, and the patients were discharged within ten days. The coloanal anastomosis was dilated daily for two to three months, and perianal excoriation resolved within six months.

Looking back at this paper by So et al, surprisingly little has changed in the surgical management of HD, although operative techniques have evolved. As rightly stated by the authors, successful colonic washouts remain the key prerequisite to avoid preliminary enterostomy, although polyethylene glycol started on the day preceding surgery has replaced prolonged bowel preparation and enteral antibiotics. While waiting for the operation, parents are nowadays thought to perform washouts at home after documentation of successful bowel decompression at hospital. Since 1980, after the mucosectomy part of endorectal pull-through was gradually transformed by several authors to take place completely through transanal route in combination with laparotomy or laparoscopy (3–5), the entire operation for rectosigmoid Hirschsprung's disease became possible through the anus following description of transanal endorectal pull-through by De la Torre (6). In line with results of So et al., the incidence of surgical complications of primary endorectal pull-through has remained low despite these technical advancements. Also, functional outcomes achieved by So et al. mirror current findings, as they reported continence rate around 80% in their follow-up paper published nearly two decades later (7).

Since publication, primary pull-through has been widely adopted across the world, representing one of the most significant advancements in surgical management of Hirschsprung's disease. One-stage operation not only reduces the number of laparotomies, but also prevents frequent enterostomy complications without jeopardising functional outcomes.

REFERENCES

1. Soave F. Hirschsprung's disease: A new surgical technique. Arch Dis Child. 1964;39:116–24.
2. Boley SJ. An endorectal pull-through operation with primary anastomosis for Hirschsprung's disease. Surg Gyn Obstet. 1968;127:353–57.
3. Rintala RJ, Lindahl H. Transanal endorectal coloanal anastomosis for Hirschsprung's disease. Pediatr Surg Int. 1993;8:128–31.
4. Georgeson KE, Fuenter MM, Hardin WD. Primary laparoscopic pull-through for Hirschsprung's disease. J Pediatr Surg. 1995;30:1017–22.
5. Saltzman DA, Telander MJ, Brennon WS, Telander RL. Transanal mucosectomy: A modification of the soave procedure for Hirschsprung's disease. J Pediatr Surg. 1996;31:1272–75.
6. De la Torre-Mondragón, Ortega-Saldugo JA. Transanal endorectal pull-through for Hirschsprung's disease. J Pediatr Surg. 1998;33:1283–86.
7. So HB, Becker JM, Schwartz, Kutin ND. Eighteen years' experience with neonatal Hirschsprung's disease treated by endorectal pull-through without colostomy. J Pediatr Surg. 1998; 33:673–675.

CHAPTER 23

Posterior Sagittal Anorectoplasty

Pieter A de Vries and Alberto Peña

Journal of Pediatric Surgery 1982; 17(5):638–643.
Citations: *n* = 421

Posterior Sagittal Anorectoplasty

By Pieter A. deVries and Alberto Peña

Kansas City, Kansas and Mexico City D.F.

ABSTRACT

The abstract simply describes the technique and provides no information on actual outcome of the operated patients. All this is contained in the body of the paper, and this describes the outcomes in a series of 34 patients (October 1980–December 1981) operated on using a new approach first described by Alberto Peña in a presentation to the Pacific Association of Pediatric Surgery (PAPS) in May 1980. Most of the patients in the series were operated on in Mexico City and were usually children, not infants. The steps of the operation are described in great detail, including midline skin incision from sacrum to perineum; midline division of the levator and striated muscle complex aided by use of an electrostimulator; and identification of the terminal intestine and fistula (if any).

As with a lot of this kind of anorectal surgery, outcomes are only loosely and subjectively described. Indeed, only 12 of the series had had their stomas closed, and of these, eight, ranging from eight months to eight years, are described as having 'excellent results', with clinical details provided in the form of a table. Likewise, the failures ranging from three to nine years of age are also detailed in a table, and of these it is noteworthy that one had a cloaca and absent sacrum and two deformed sacra.

Operative photographs are reprinted, but as these are in black and white, they don't add too much to visual understanding.

This paper was based on a presentation to the Surgical Section of the American Academy of Pediatrics (October, 1981).

DOI: 10.1201/9781003341901-23

COMMENTARY (MARK DAVENPORT)

This operation was a radical departure for paediatric surgeons of the day. Most had been brought up on the teachings of Douglas Stephens from Melbourne, who, based on a large series of postmortem dissections of children with anorectal malformations (ARM) in the early 1950s, advocated a relatively blind approach for high anorectal malformations, using a small incision near the coccyx to identify the distal rectum and the creation of a tunnel by feel, through the puborectalis muscle sling in front of the urethra (1). Peña's approach evolved during the 1970s, ultimately extending this posterior incision and dividing striated muscle fibres to actually visualise the components of the anomaly.

Pieter de Vries, a paediatric surgeon from Sacramento, California, was the other author on these papers, and the two first met in March 1980 at a PAPS meeting and subsequently operated together. However, that first paper was submitted without Peña's knowledge, and this caused a substantial rift between the two (2).

Posterior Sagittal Anorectoplasty: Important Technical Considerations and New Applications

By Alberto Peña and Pieter A. Devries
Mexico City

The follow-up paper published only two months later in the same journal, with the authors' names now reversed, described 54 patients and was Peña's own work (3). This too arose from presentation to the thirteenth American Pediatric Surgical Association (APSA) meeting in May 1982 (Figure 23.2). I think today we would probably not accept such duplication of content in both meetings and publications! Again, there is more focus on the technique than the results, with extra details of the separation of rectum from the urethra and the tapering of the pulled-through dilated ectatic rectum. The paper provides 15 figures including details of individual cases, particularly cloacas. Interestingly, the meeting's discussion is also given with some support shown, though there were also some sceptics, notably John Raffensperger from Chicago.

Raffensperger notwithstanding, the technique of posterior sagital anorectoplasty (PSARP) was taken up with enthusiasm throughout the world, undoubtedly aided by Alberto Peña's constant touring and willingness to demonstrate his operation in meetings and symposia wherever they may be.

Peña's interpretation of the anatomy and pathology of ARM also gained more traction with more and more surgeons being influenced by his operation. He was central to the adoption of the Krickenbeck classification. This was based on an international meeting in Germany in 2005 (4), replacing the older Wingspread classification, itself based on an international meeting in Wisconsin in 1984.

REFERENCES

1. Stephens FD. Imperforate rectum. A new surgical technique. Med J Aust. 1953;1:202–3.
2. Peña A. The story of the posterior saggital approach. In: Monologues of a Pediatric Surgeon. 2011, pp. 83–134.
3. Peña A, Devries PA. Posterior sagittal anorectoplasty: Important technical considerations and new applications. J Pediatr Surg. 1982;17(6):796–811.
4. Holschneider A, Hutson J, Peña A, et al. preliminary report on the international conference for the development of standards for the treatment of anorectal malformations. J Pediatr Surg. 2005;40:1521–6.

CHAPTER 24

Preliminary Report on the International Conference for the Development of Standards for the Treatment of Anorectal Malformations

Alexander Holschneider, John Hutson, Albert Peña,
Elhamy Beket et al. (+ 22 others)

Journal of Pediatric Surgery 2005; 40:1521–1526.
Citations: $n = 435$

ABSTRACT

Background: Anorectal malformations (ARM) are common congenital anomalies seen throughout the world. Comparison of outcome data has been hindered because of confusion related to classification and assessment systems.

Methods: The goals of the Krickenbeck Conference on ARM was to develop standards for an international classification of ARM based on a modification of fistula type and adding rare and regional variants, and to design a system for comparable follow-up studies.

Results: Lesions were classified into major clinical groups based on the fistula location (perineal, recto-urethral, rectovesical, vestibular), cloacal lesions, those with no fistula and anal stenosis. Rare and regional variants included pouch colon, rectal atresia or stenosis, rectovaginal fistula, H-fistula and others. Groups would be analysed according to the type of procedure performed stratified for confounding associated conditions such as sacral anomalies and tethered cord. A standard method for postoperative assessment of continence was determined.

Conclusions: A new international diagnostic classification system, operative groupings and a method of postoperative assessment of continence were developed by consensus of a large contingent of participants experienced in the management of patients with ARM. These methods should allow for a common standardisation of diagnosis and comparing postoperative results.

DOI: 10.1201/9781003341901-24

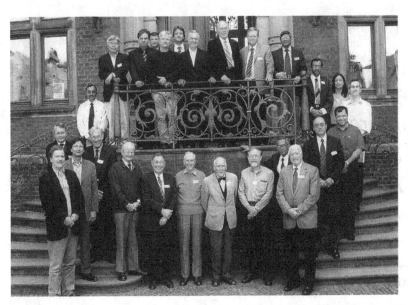

Figure 24.1   *Group photograph from Krinkenbeck (from paper)*. (Reprinted with permission from Elsevier, 'Preliminary report on the International Conference for the Development of Standards for the Treatment of Anorectal Malformations', Alexander Holschneider, John Hutson, Albert Peña, Elhamy Beket et al. (+22 others), Journal of Pediatric Surgery 2005; 40: 1521–1526. https://doi.org/10.1016/j.jpedsurg.2005.08.002.)

COMMENTARY (RISTO RINTALA)

This was based on an international congress for the development of standards for the treatment of anorectal malformations and was organised in Krickenbeck Castle, near Dusseldorf, Germany, in May 17–20, 2005, by Professor Alexander Holschneider of Cologne. The aim of the meeting was to develop a practical clinical classification, standards for the treatment and a follow-up scoring system for anorectal malformations. The previous widely accepted classifications, the International Classification of Anorectal Malformations from the early 1970s and the Wingspread classification of anorectal malformations from 1984 (1) that distinguished between high, intermediate and low malformations in both sexes, were considered too detailed and difficult to use in clinical practice. Moreover, knowledge of surgical anatomy of anorectal malformations and operative techniques had been revolutionised by the work of Alberto Peña and Pieter deVries and their concept of posterior sagittal anorectoplasty (PSARP). Twenty-six authorities on pediatric colorectal and pelvic disorders from all over the world were invited to this meeting, including the main figures in the background of the previous classifications, F. Douglas Stephens and Durham Smith from Australia (Figure 24.1).

The conference was a consensus meeting. During the sessions, the classification, surgical treatment and principles of follow-up were widely discussed by the participants. A new classification was proposed, and this was largely based on the classification of Alberto Peña from 1995 (2). The new practical classification was based on major clinical groups that were characterised by the type of the fistula. Rare and regional variants of anorectal malformations were included in the classification.

The proposed new classification of postoperative outcomes was based on the presence of voluntary bowel movements, soiling and constipation. This simple and descriptive scoring system raised a lot of discussion as there were preexisting outcome scoring systems that gave a clear numerical score that could be used in comparative and statistical analyses. The proceedings and discussions during the Krickenbeck consensus conference created a basis for the book *Anorectal Malformations in Children* that was published 2006 by Springer.

In the beginning the results of the Krickenbeck conference did not impact significantly the pediatric surgical literature. Wingspread classification and various outcome scores continued to be in use in numerous publications. The practicality and simplicity of the Krickenbeck classification have gradually emerged in the research on anorectal malformations and undoubtedly is today the classification that is best for comparison of clinical and follow-up studies. The Krickenbeck scoring of outcomes is also widely used, but its descriptive nature and lack of numerical score points diminish its comparability. The third aim of the conference, developing standards for the treatment of anorectal malformations, was not as successful as the classifications. While the PSARP is still the 'gold standard' for the surgical treatment, mini-invasive and hybrid techniques have emerged especially for the management of more severe anorectal malformations.

REFERENCES

1. Smith ED, Stephens FD, Holschneider AM, Nixon HH, Peña A. Operations to improve continence after previous surgery. Birth Defects Orig Artic Ser. 1988;24(4):447–79.
2. Peña A. Anorectal malformations. Semin Pediatr Surg. 1995;4:35–47.

CHAPTER 25

A New Operation for Non-Correctable Biliary Atresia: Hepatic Portoenterostomy. (In Japanese)

Morio Kasai, Munezo Suzuki

Shujutsu [Surgical Operation]. 1959; 13:733–739.
Citations: not known

ABSTRACT

This paper describes the first 12 patients in the evolution of what became known as the Kasai portoenterostomy. All the operations were performed at Tohoku University Hospital in Sendai, on the east coast of Japan. It begins with a review of the history of surgery in biliary atresia (BA) and a table of 12 previous reports (11 being in English starting with Holmes in 1916 (1)). This paper had reviewed the literature to that date and suggested a 16% restoration of bile flow. All subsequent communications had emphasised the dismal outcomes of any attempt.

Four of the early operations, starting in 1953, were done by the chief of surgery at that time, Dr Katsura, with Dr Kasai taking over for the rest. The first case was operated on at 150 days but died of respiratory problems in the early postoperative period. The second case, in 1955, was a child with Turner syndrome. During dissection in the porta hepatis trying to find residual biliary structures, they encountered significant bleeding. They placed the incised duodenum up to the porta hepatis and later were astonished at the reappearance of bile pigment in the stool and a fall in serum bilirubin. She proved to be a long-term survivor (Sendai records suggest her being alive at the age of 38 years). The third case was probably not type III and had a nonincised duodenum attached to the porta hepatis. She died at the age of seven months. The postmortem showed the development of an internal bilioenteric fistula between the duodenum and porta hepatis. The fourth case is probably the most remarkable. She had type I cyst and had the duodenum anastomosed to the transected cyst, leaving the gallbladder *in situ*. She was a long-term survivor, ultimately dying of cholangiocarcinoma at age 63 years (2).

Eight other cases were described, and, from 1957, the authors changed from using the duodenum or stomach to creating a Roux loop with mobilised jejunum (Figure 25.1) for the last four.

   DOI: 10.1201/9781003341901-25

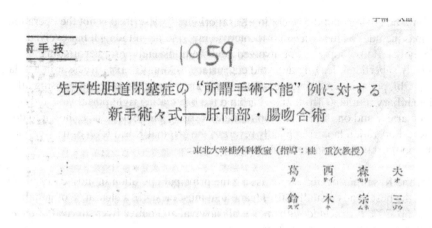

Figure 25.1 Original 1959 Shujutsu paper in Japanese.

Histological appreciation of the resected en-bloc proximal biliary remnant was also detailed and showed a myriad of microscopic biliary ductules within, with the presumption that these communicated with intrahepatic ducts. This was an important scientific observation reinforcing the credentials of what Kasai was writing about.

COMMENTARY (MARK DAVENPORT WITH MAJOR ASSISTANCE FROM ATSUYUKI YAMATAKA AND MASAKI NIO)

This Japanese paper describes something that is not uncommon in medicine being facilitated by the unintended consequences of doing something different. Though not described in detail in the abstract, the chief of surgery in 1955 in Sendai was a Dr Katsura, and he doesn't even get his name on the paper! Their third case was problematic, with on-table bleeding, not surprising given she was 72 days old at time of surgery. They placed the incised duodenum up to the porta hepatis to try and staunch this, were successful and then later were astonished at the reappearance of bile pigment in the stool and a fall in serum bilirubin.

Dr Kasai reported this new operative technique in 1959 (2) and then in German in 1963 and finally in English in 1968 (3). However, the merits of this surgery were slowly appreciated by surgeons outside of Japan, and it was only during the 1970s that surgeons in Europe and North America started to perform it, often following a visit to Sendai to watch the maestro Kasai in action.

Nevertheless, it is important to realise that the results from this early experience were not good, and in a later paper (4) it was reported that only three (12%) of this early series to 1961 ($n = 21$) actually cleared their jaundice, and of these two survived long term.

It should be obvious but the operation Kasai originally described is not the operation that masquerades as the 'Kasai portoenterostomy' operation today. It has evolved. Originally a Roux loop was not involved, and the transected porta hepatis was relatively superficial, leaving an ovoid cut surface to join. Kasai's successor in Sendai, Riyoji Ohi, pursued a more aggressive approach to the porta dissection excising all visible biliary remnants from in and around the bifurcating right portal vein and right hepatic artery and on the left side up to the Rex fossa. Those who have chosen to do the Kasai operation laparoscopically revert to the original Kasai level of transection with good outcomes in some hands (5).

Today the Kasai portoenterostomy is still the principal operation in most cases of BA, and in the best hands (usually still Japanese, it must be said), a clearance of jaundice rate of 60–70% is expected with an overall survival and native liver survival of 89% and 49% at 20 years, respectively (6).

REFERENCES

1. Holmes JB. Congenital obliteration of the bile ducts: Diagnosis and suggestions for treatment. Am J Dis Child. 1916;11:405.
2. Nio M, Wada M, Sasaki H, et al. Correctable biliary atresia and cholangiocarcinoma: A case report of a 63-year-old patient. Surgical Case Reports. 2019;5:185.
3. Kasai M, Kimura S, Asakura Y, Suzuki H, et al. Surgical treatment of biliary atresia. J Pediatr Surg. 1968; 3:665.
4. Ohi R. History of the Kasai operation: Hepatic portoenterostomy for biliary atresia. World J Surg. 1988;12:871–74.
5. Koga H, Miyano G, Takahashi T, Shimotakahara A, Kato Y, et al. Laparoscopic portoenterostomy for uncorrectable biliary atresia using Kasai's original technique. J Laparoendosc Adv Surg Tech A. 2011;21:291–94.
6. Nio M. Japanese biliary atresia registry. Pediatr Surg Int. 2017;33(12):1319–25.

CHAPTER 26

Congenital Bile Duct Cysts Classification, Operative Procedures, and Review of Thirty-Seven Cases Including Cancer Arising from Choledochal Cyst

Todani T, Watanabe Y, Narusue M, Tabuchi K, and Okajlma K

American Journal of Surgery 1977; 134(2):263–269.
doi: 10.1016/0002-9610(77)90359-2.
Citations: $n = 1,161$

ABSTRACT

Thirty-seven patients with congenital bile duct cysts, including 17 children and nine young adults, were encountered from 1960 to April 1976. Since the congenital bile duct cysts were observed in many parts of the bile duct, from the liver to the duodenum, we prefer to use the term 'bile duct cyst', and we classify these cysts into

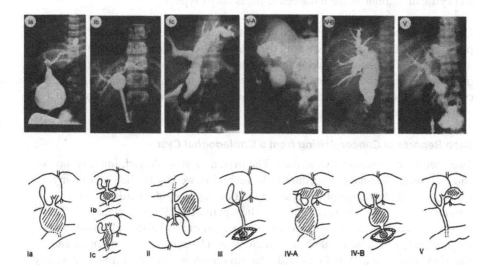

Figure 26.1 Top: typical operative cholangiograms of congenital bile duct cysts: from left to right, types Ia, common type; Ib segmental dilatation; Ic, diffuse dilatation; IV-A multiple cyst (intra- and extrahepatic); types IV-B, multiple cyst (extrahepatic only); and V, intrahepatic cysts. Bottom: associated diagrams demonstrating typing of ductal cysts: from left to right, types Ia, Ib, Ic, II, III, IV-A, IV-B and V. (Courtesy of Elsevier.)

six types for surgical treatment, in contrast with Alonso-Lej's classification. Based on experience with two patients in whom cancer arose from a choledochal cyst, it seems that excision of the choledochal cyst is always the most desirable operation for Type Ia and Ib cysts in older children and young adults. Partial resection of intrahepatic cysts should be added in some cases of type IV-A cysts to achieve free drainage of the bile juice from the intrahepatic cysts.

COMMENTARY (MARK DAVENPORT)

This is a remarkable paper from a relatively small city, Okayamaon on Honshu, the southern island of Japan, about 410 miles from Tokyo. All the major advances during this period in this disease were occurring in Japan, partly due of course to the Asian predisposition to choledochal malformations and it being relatively rare in the West.

This series was used as the basis for modification of a previous comprehensive review and classification published in 1959 by American surgeons Alonso-Lej, Rever and Pessagno (1). In turn, it was based upon the published literature to date of about 100 cases and divided choledochal cysts in three types: I, extrahepatic; II, diverticulum; and III, choledochoceles (localised dilatation of the bile duct as it entered the wall of the duodenum). Seventeen patients in the Todani series, all with extrahepatic dilatation, could fit into the Alonso-Lej classification, but crucially 20 could not. So, 15 had an additional intrahepatic cyst (now reclassified as Type IV-A), one had multiple cystic dilatations in the extrahepatic bile duct (Type IVB) and four had cystic dilatations in the intrahepatic ducts only (Type V).

Operative procedures were described for all the cases and reflected the surgical philosophy of the day. So, this was in the form of external drainage ($n = 3$); internal drainage ($n = 17$) (mainly choledochocystoduodenostomy); and cyst excision ($n = 13$) (mainly hepaticoduodenostomy) for the Type I and IV cysts. The remaining Type V cysts were treated either by partial hepatectomy ($n = 3$) or internal drainage with a choledochojejunostomy Roux-en-Y.

Case Reports of Cancer Arising from a Choledochal Cyst

Two specific patients were described. The first, a 17-year-old girl, initially having had an internal drainage procedure at 14 years followed by further laparotomy which showed shrinkage of the cyst but the development of a hard, polypoid tumour on the posterior wall – shown to be squamous cell carcinoma. She died shortly after a definitive resection. The second patient had also undergone biliary surgery earlier that included cholecystectomy at 15 years, but re-presented and was shown to have a Type IV choledochal dilatation which was drained internally to the duodenum. Reexploration was later performed, and the patient was shown to have a large 'cancerous tumour' with multiple liver metastases and died shortly afterwards.

Classification

The authors proposed changing this by expanding Type I to include (A) classical extrahepatic choledochal cyst, (B) segmental choledochal dilatation and (C) diffuse or cylindrical dilatation (now commonly termed 'fusiform'); by subdividing Type IV as (A), both extra- and intrahepatic dilatation or (B) multiple cysts within extrahepatic duct and Type V as intrahepatic dilatation only.

Cancer

In addition to their own cases, they reviewed 36 previously published cases and use this to push strongly for excision and biliary reconstruction as the definitive operation rather than leaving residual tissue, which may still be the focus for recurrent inflammation and infection predisposing to malignant transformation.

The series was made possible by the increasing use of operative cholangiography, not available to earlier authors. They realised the nuances of extrahepatic dilatation, recognising some which did not have the typical classic cyst appearance, though never mentioning any relationship with the distal arrangement of the bile duct with pancreatic duct. They inferred that Type IV cysts were a natural development of a preexisting extrahepatic dilatation occurring in older children and adults.

There is a disconnect of some of the cholangiographic examples of each type with its schematic in Figure 26.1. So, the Type V case as illustrated has a far from normal common bile duct, and the Type IVB similarly has gross intrahepatic dilatation accompanying it.

The paper was also influential in moving surgeons away from simple internal drainage operations, which admittedly cure the jaundice but leave lots of potential for future problems (including cancer) with undrained segments of cyst in direct communication typically with the duodenum. Where they backed the wrong horse was in persisting with a hepaticoduodenostomy biliary reconstruction rather than a hepaticojejunostomy Roux-en-Y. Takuji Todani, a prolific author in this field, continued with this approach for the rest of his career, only stopping when a cancer occurred 19 years after excision and hepaticoduodenostomy when the child was only one year old (2). Somewhat ironically, hepaticoduodenostomy for reconstruction has made a comeback as an easier alternative to the Roux loop for laparoscopic reconstruction.

This series doesn't mention or try to explain aetiology of these 'bile duct cysts' – their preferred term – leaving that to other Japanese groups. At King's College Hospital, we became interested in the aetiological aspects of *choledochal malformation* – our preferred term – during the 1990s and developed our own simplified modification of the Todani classification (3). We only really recognised the cystic and fusiform variants of Type I (Type 1 C and 1 F respectively) and using the same concept for Type IV (Type 4C and 4F), showing pathophysiological differences of intraductal pressure and pancreatic reflux between them. Latterly it has also become clear that Type V lesions can be independent of the features of Caroli's disease or syndrome. This really is a separate entity to all the foregoing with a fundamental defect in intrahepatic bile duct basement membrane integrity with diminution in laminin and Type IV collagen both in the liver and kidney and an intrinsic tendency to severe liver and renal fibrosis respectively.

REFERENCES

1. Alonso-Lej F, Rever WH, Pessagno DJ. Congenital choledochal cyst, with a report of 2 and an analysis of 94, cases. Int Abstr Surg. 1959;108:1–30.
2. Todani T, Watanabe Y, Toki A, Hara H. Hilar duct carcinoma developed after cyst excision followed by hepaticoduodenostomy. In: Koyanagi Y, Aoki T (eds) Pancreaticobiliary Maljunction. Igaku Tosho Shuppan, Tokyo; 2002:17–21.
3. Kronfli R, Davenport M. Insights into the pathophysiology and classification of type 4 choledochal malformation. J Pediatr Surg. 2020;55(12):2642–46.

CHAPTER 27

Seamless Management of Biliary Atresia in England and Wales (1999–2002)

Mark Davenport, Jean De Ville de Goyet, Mark D Stringer,
Giorgina Mieli-Vergani, Deirdre A Kelly, Pat McClean, and Lewis Spitz

The Lancet 2004 April 24; 363(9418):1354–1357.
Citations: $n = 233$

ABSTRACT

This series describes the early outcome of a national (England and Wales) policy change in the management of biliary atresia (BA) from a decentralised one based on regional neonatal surgical centres (potentially $n = 25$) to one based on specialist hepatobiliary centres co-locating facilities for the Kasai operation and liver transplantation ($n = 3$).

One hundred forty-eight infants with BA were treated between January 1999 and June 2002. A primary Kasai portoenterostomy was done in 142 (96%) infants and a primary liver transplant in five (3%). One child died before any intervention. Early clearance of jaundice (defined as achieving a bilirubin of < 20 µmol/L) after Kasai was achieved in 81 of 142 (57%) infants. Liver transplantation was done in 52 (37%) of those undergoing Kasai. Thirteen (9%) infants died.

Of the 135 children who survived, 84 (62%) still have their native liver and 51 (38%) had transplantation. The median follow-up of survivors was 2·13 (range 0·5–4·1) years. The overall four-year estimated actuarial survival was 89% (95% CI 82–94). The four-year estimated actuarial survival with native liver was 51% (42–59%).

COMMENTARY (MARK DAVENPORT)

The outcome of management of BA has been a subject of great scrutiny, out of all proportion to its actual frequency in the population. This was more so in the UK with two national surveys of practice in the 1980s and 1990s (1, 2). Both showed the same thing, that where you were treated was important and specifically if that centre treated more than five patients a year, then chances of survival improved markedly. The government of the day, led by Tony Blair, had already been stung by a media outcry following the revelations of the Bristol heart surgery scandal in infants with transposition of the great vessels and didn't want to go down the same route. So, from 1999, they restricted management of BA to only three English units – King's College Hospital in London, and children's hospitals in Birmingham and Leeds. This happened despite much wailing and gnashing of teeth from those children's hospitals excluded from the process such as those in Liverpool and Manchester (3, 4).

This series showed that following this change, good results (more than comparable to published results from Europe and North America) could be obtained when rolled out on a national basis and was later confirmed when the ten-year results became available in 2011 (5). As time marched on, children from the other UK nations, Scotland and Northern Ireland, also fell in with this policy, and then from about 2010 the same thing happened when the Republic of Ireland started referring their infants across the Irish Sea. This centralisation strategy for BA was also adopted by Scandinavian countries such as Finland, Sweden, Denmark and Norway and some northern European countries such as the Netherlands, Poland and most recently even Germany (6).

Centralisation as a concept can of course be applied to other aspects of surgery, specifically paediatric surgery, where the cases are usually few and far between and surgical expertise and experience makes a difference to outcome. In the UK, this strategy has been adopted for the management of bladder exstrophy with many also calling for the management of long-gap and isolated oesophageal atresia to be restricted to only a few centres. Health providers in the Netherlands have also rearranged services using these principles for paediatric oncology, where there is now only a single centre and not in the capital or one of the two major Dutch cities Amsterdam or Rotterdam but in Utrecht (7).

REFERENCES

1. McClement JW, Howard ER, Mowat AP. Results of surgical treatment for extrahepatic biliary atresia in United Kingdom 1980-2. Survey conducted on behalf of the British Paediatric Association Gastroenterology Group and the British Association of Paediatric Surgeons. Br Med J (Clin Res Ed). 1985;290(6465):345–47.
2. McKiernan PJ, Baker AJ, Kelly DA. The frequency and outcome of biliary atresia in the UK and Ireland. Lancet. 2000;355(9197):25–29.
3. Davison S, Miller V, Thomas A, Bowen J, Bruce J. The profession, not the media, should assess where Kasai portoenterostomy should be performed. BMJ. 1999;318:1013
4. Lloyd D, Jones M, Dalzell M. Surgery for biliary atresia. Lancet. 2000;355:1099–1100.
5. Davenport M, Ong E, Sharif K, et al. Biliary atresia in England and Wales: results of centralization and new benchmark. J Pediatr Surg. 2011;46(9):1689–94.
6. Lampela H, Ritvanen A, Kosola S, et al. National centralization of biliary atresia care to an assigned multidisciplinary team provides high-quality outcomes. Scand J Gastroenterol. 2012;47(1):99–107. doi: 10.3109/00365521.2011.627446. PMID: 22171974.
7. Wijnen MH, Hulscher JB. Centralization of pediatric surgical care in the Netherlands: Lessons learned. J Pediatr Surg. 2022;57(2):178–181.

CHAPTER 28

Gastroschisis: A Simple Technique for Staged Silo Closure

James D Fischer, Karen Chun, Donald C Moores, and H Gibbs Andrews

Journal of Pediatric Surgery 1995; 30(8):1169–1171.
Citations: *n* = 69

ABSTRACT

The authors report their initial use of a preformed spring-loaded silicone rubber silo (Silastic®) bag (Figure 28.1) to cover the eviscerated gut in infants with gastroschisis. This was applied by the cot-side on the neonatal unit with the help of a sedative agent (Fentanyl). The eviscerated intestines were then gradually reduced over a number of days before formal surgical fascial closure was performed. Initially, this was undertaken in the operating room; however, later in the series cot-side silo removal and fascial closure under sedation was successful.

From October 1992 to April 1994, the authors managed ten infants using this protocol. The results were compared with gastroschisis infants treated conventionally between August 1982 and June 1993. Though there was no actual statistical comparison, outcome measures such as time to full closure (range: two to eight days), time to full enteral nutrition (range: 11–25 days) and time to discharge (range 12–37 days) seemed similar.

The procedure was well tolerated in the ten infants and there was no incidence of bowel injury, dehiscence of the closure, sepsis or necrotizing enterocolitis.

COMMENTARY (BASHAR ALDEIRI)

This report from Loma Linda Children's Hospital in California started a new era in the management of infants with gastroschisis. Until then, the mainstay of gastroschisis management was primary surgical fascial closure under general anesthesia. When this was not feasible, a custom-made silo typically made out of silicone sheets or nonabsorbable mesh was constructed to allow staged visceral reduction and delayed fascial closure.

The application of a preformed silo (PFS), almost universally (with exceptions for closed gastroschisis etc.), from the outset offered many advantages in the management of gastroschisis such as early coverage of the eviscerated bowel at the cot side; continuous monitoring of the herniated viscera with gradual reduction in order

DOI: 10.1201/9781003341901-28

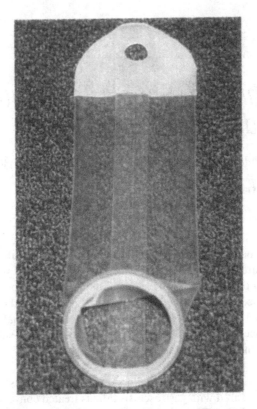

Figure 28.1   Silastic® silo with spring-loaded ring. (Courtesy of Elsevier.)

to develop an abdominal domain, and avoidance of out-of-hours anaesthesia in a just-born infant. It was not long before many pediatric surgeons in North America embraced the new technique and adopted it in their routine practice with enthusiasm (1). Thereafter, it crossed the Atlantic and has received wide recognition globally (1, 2). The practice of cot-side silo application, removal and a sutureless gastroschisis closure is now the preferred option in many units. Nonetheless, actual differences in outcome compared to the traditional approach remain elusive, and a systematic review of literature published up to 2014 found very little concrete differences (3).

This wasn't the first report of this principle. That honour should perhaps go to a report published over 20 years previously by Dennis Shermeta and Alex Haller Jr. from Johns Hopkins, Baltimore. They used the term 'preformed silo' in 1975 (4) in a series of nine infants with gastroschisis. The authors applied a bespoke transparent silicone bag over the eviscerated bowel; this was then secured in place by inserting an attached compressible silicone polymer ring inside the abdomen. The silicone ring was sutured to the fascia for extra security and to prevent accidental silo displacement. The preformed silo was held in an upright position in the infant's cot, while gradually reducing the eviscerated contents. The silo was then removed and formal surgical closure of the fascial defect took place 9–12 days from the initial insertion. Why this prototype of preformed silo failed to gain popularity is not known. Certainly, the paper was not quoted by Fischer et al.

REFERENCES

1. Aldrink JH, Caniano DA, Nwomeh BC. Variability in gastroschisis management: A survey of North American pediatric surgery training programs. J Surg Res. 2012;176(1):159–63.
2. Zani A, Ruttenstock E, Davenport M, Ade-Ajayi N. Is there unity in Europe? First survey of EUPSA delegates on the management of gastroschisis. Eur J Pediatr Surg. 2013;23:19–24.
3. Shermeta DW, Haller JA Jr. A new preformed transparent silo for the management of gastroschisis. J Pediatr Surg. 1975;10(6):973–75.
4. Ross AR, Eaton S, Zani A, et al. The role of preformed silos in the management of infants with gastroschisis: A systematic review and meta-analysis. Pediatr Surg Int. 2015;31(5):473–83.

CHAPTER 29

Gastroschisis: A National Cohort Study to Describe Contemporary Surgical Strategies and Outcomes

Owen A, Marven S, Johnson P, Kurinczuk J, Spark P, Draper ES, Brocklehurst P, Knight M; BAPS-CASS

Journal of Pediatric Surgery 2010; 45(9):1808–1816.
Citations: $n = 78$

ABSTRACT

This was a survey of all the cases of gastroschisis ($n = 393$) managed within the 28 neonatal surgical units in the UK and Ireland (18 months in 2006–2008) from a predicted birth cohort of 1.1 million.

Results: Infants were divided into simple gastroschisis ($n = 336$, 85.5%) and complex gastroschisis ($n = 45$, 11.5%) – unknown category ($n = 12$, 3%). Virtually all were detected antenatally ($n = 385$, 98%).

Operative primary closure ($n = 170$, 51%) and staged closure after a preformed silo ($n = 120$, 36%) were the most commonly used techniques by intension for simple gastroschisis.

There were 6 (2%) neonatal deaths (all in the simple group). Outcomes for infants in the complex group were significantly worse. They were more likely to be ventilated postoperatively (risk ratio [RR], 1.21; 95% CI, 1.09–1.33), more likely to require reoperation (RR, 6.53; 95% CI, 4.70–9.09), more likely to develop intestinal failure associated liver disease (RR, 8.21; 95% CI, 3.70–18.2) and more likely to receive total parenteral nutrition for >28 days (RR, 2.07; 95% CI, 1.71–2.51).

Conclusions: This study provided a comprehensive picture of current UK and Ireland practice for gastroschisis and a national benchmark.

COMMENTARY (SEAN MARVEN)

We had become interested in strategies for reduction and closure of gastroschisis in the midst of an apparent epidemic of gastroschisis in the UK and Ireland.

DOI: 10.1201/9781003341901-29

I returned from a three-month trip to the Rocky Mountain Children's Hospital in Denver with some samples of the 'spring-loaded silo' in 2001. Unfortunately, 9/11 put a stop to any further supplies. A trout fishing trip to Ireland led to a serendipitous collaboration with a British medical company, Medicina, that kindly established the production of my design for a preformed entirely silicone-based silo. Successful reduction and closure of 21 patients without general anaesthetic or postoperative ventilation was presented to the British Association of Paediatric Surgeons (BAPS) in Dublin in 2005 and published thereafter in the *Journal of Pediatric Surgery* in 2006 (1).

We felt that it ought to be possible to look at outcomes in the UK of different strategies and to see how the diffusion of this disruptive new technology was progressing. Was there a superior technique?

At the time, there was not much new in gastroschisis research. Parenteral nutrition was life-saving, but potentially harmful. Operative primary reduction and fascial closure was considered the gold standard. Adrian Bianchi's novel cot-side method (2) was not as easy as it sounded, and custom-sutured silos were still required in nearly half of all cases. We sensed not all cases were equal, but that the intention to treat nonoperatively was pivotal.

The superiority of any strategy was not apparent at this stage. Was the preformed silo just turning the clock back? Did it meet the needs of non-co-located maternity and surgical units with resource limitations? Or, did it offer to minimise the need to operate in the middle of the night? In many ways, it made good sense to perform a gradual physiological reduction with bedside closure. This together with the avoidance of general anaesthesia d and minimising the risk of abdominal compartment syndrome, became the cornerstones of the technique. We were happily unconscious of how important the 'sutureless' defect closure was in facilitating complete reduction and limiting increase of intra-abdominal pressure.

The pendulum between primary and staged reduction seemed to be swinging back and forth over the decades. Publication of an array of surrogate outcome measures was focused largely on surgical parameters from single institutions.

The UK and Ireland at the time were incompletely covered by regional congenital anomaly registers. Our ideas for a national study led to a collaboration with the Oxford-based National Perinatal Epidemiology Unit and foundation of the BAPS Congenital Anomaly Surveillance System (BAPS-CASS), led by the indomitable Marion Knight and her team.

And so surveillance postcards were distributed to every centre and returned notifying cases, and the data were analysed in Oxford. A population-based cohort study of all live-born infants with gastroschisis born in the UK and Ireland from October 2006 to March 2008 was completed. It all seemed so easy, but in reality, it was a difficult birth.

It did seem to stimulate other large datasets and population cohorts in other countries. It also contributed to the call for national registries for congenital anomalies. Perhaps most importantly, it initiated and embedded the idea of collaborative research by the paediatric surgeons in the UK and Ireland, who historically did not usually suffer from equipoise.

We were initially unaware how much it would polarise thinking. However, subsequently the idea permeated to low- and middle-income countries and gained traction with a Welcome Funded study offering the possibility of survival where gastroschisis was almost uniformly fatal (3).

Meanwhile, the debate still rages, the pendulum still swings and more data on outcomes emerge (4, 5). It seems likely that attempted primary reduction with sutured closure in daylight and within three hours of birth might be the optimal first intention for inborn babies. But perhaps the practical reality is a local surgical pathway where either option may be the primary intention, according to resources and / or risk categorisation.

COMMENTARY (MARK DAVENPORT)

The BAPS-CASS was a collaboration between Oxford obstetric epidemiologists led by Marian Knight and the national organisation of UK and Irish paediatric surgeons (BAPS) to determine snapshots of outcomes of several common neonatal surgical conditions, such as diaphragmatic hernias, posterior urethral valves etc. This paper was the first in this series. It is remarkable in that it is comprehensive national dataset that actually does not conclude on what is the best of a range of possible surgical options for the condition. The use of a preformed silo had just been introduced into UK practice but was becoming more widespread (about 1/3 of simple cases), though operative primary fascial closure was still the most popular option (just over half of cases).

There was a one-year follow-up study published the following year (6) which extended the results, noting six more deaths with a mortality rate therefore of 4% and had an increased citation rate (*n* = 48), possibly because it was in a higher impact generalist journal (*British Medical Journal*).

REFERENCES

1. Owen A, Marven S, Jackson L, et al. Experience of bedside preformed silo staged reduction and closure for gastroschisis. J Pediatr Surg. 2006;41(11):1830–35.
2. Bianchi A, Dickson AP. Elective delayed reduction and no anesthesia: 'minimal intervention management' for gastroschisis. J Pediatr Surg. 1998;33:1338–40.
3. Wright N, Abantanga F, Amoah M, et al. Developing and implementing an interventional bundle to reduce mortality from gastroschisis in low-resource settings. Wellcome Open Res. 2019;4:46. doi: 10.12688/wellcomeopenres.15113.1.

4. Charlesworth P, Akinnola I, Hammerton C, Praveena P, Desai A, Patel S, Davenport M. Preformed silos versus traditional abdominal wall closure in gastroschisis: 163 infants at a single institution. Eur J Pediatr Surg. 2014;24(1):88–93. doi: 10.1055/s-0033-1357755. Epub 2013 Oct 25. PMID: 24163195.
5. Ross AR, Eaton S, Zani A, Ade-Ajayi N, Pierro A, Hall NJ. The role of preformed silos in the management of infants with gastroschisis: A systematic review and meta-analysis. Pediatr Surg Int. 2015;31(5):473–83. doi: 10.1007/s00383-015-3691-2. Epub 2015 Mar 11. PMID: 25758783.
6. Bradnock TJ, Marven S, Owen A, Johnson P, Kurinczuk JJ, Spark P, Draper ES, Knight M; BAPS-CASS. Gastroschisis: One year outcomes from national cohort study. BMJ. 2011;343:d6749. doi: 10.1136/bmj.d6749. PMID: 22089731; PMCID: PMC3216470.

CHAPTER 30

Congenital Diaphragmatic Hernia in 120 Infants Treated Consecutively with Permissive Hypercapnea/Spontaneous Respiration/Elective Repair

Judd Boloker, David A Bateman, Jen-Tien Wung, and Charles JH Stolar

Journal of Pediatric Surgery 2002; 37:357–366.
Citations: $n = 374$

ABSTRACT

Introduction: Infants with congenital diaphragmatic hernia (CDH) are medically challenging to manage because of lung hypoplasia and pulmonary hypertension. The authors reported their experience using a new strategy of 'permissive hypercapnea/ spontaneous respiration' combined with delayed elective repair.

Methods: Retrospective single-center cohort study (August 1992 to February 2000).

Results: One hundred twenty consecutive infants were reviewed (inborn, $n = 67$; outborn, $n = 53$). Eighteen of 120 were regarded as exclusions and not treated (lethal anomalies $n = 6$; 'overwhelming pulmonary hypoplasia' $n = 10$; prerepair ECMO-related neurocomplications $n = 4$ – N.B.; *there is a disparity with numbers in the text*). Using this novel preoperative management approach 101/120 (84%) survived to have a surgical intervention and 91 (90%) of those survived to discharge, giving an overall survival rate of 91 (75.8%). Two survivors discharged on oxygen later died at four and seven months.

ECMO was used in 16 (13.3%). Non-ECMO ancillary treatments had no impact on survival. Surgery was transabdominal, and prosthetic patches were used in 7%. Tube thoracostomy was rare. Every inborn patient ($n = 11$) requiring a chest tube for pneumothorax died. Surgical repair of CDH was performed at an average of 98 and 118 hours for inborn and outborn survivors respectively.

Retrospective analysis of the maximum preoperative positive inspiratory pressure (PIP) used to ventilate survivors showed that increasing PIP > 26 cmH$_2$O in inborn infants did not achieve any improvement in the number of survivals.

DOI: 10.1201/9781003341901-30

Due to the low-pressure ventilation strategy applied, an oxygenation index (OI) of > 20 at six hours of life was used to identify inborn patients at high risk for mortality. All infants with an OI < 20 survived ($n = 37$), and none required ECMO. Those with an OI $\geq$ 20 ($n = 25$) showed an 80% mortality (20/25), and two of the survivors required ECMO. The six-hour OI of $\geq$ 20 showed positive predictive value for mortality of 80%.

COMMENTARY (BASHAR ALDEIRI)

This was quite a long, complicated report from the New York/Presbyterian Children's Hospital of a distinctive management approach for infants born with CDH. The series is also unusual for an American series because of its relatively low use of ECMO, something justified in the recorded comments to the floor at the end of the paper.

The authors challenged longstanding notions in ventilator management of CDH. Formerly, hyperventilation, often using high pressures, was used in an attempt to drive down CO_2 levels and achieve a measure of alkalinisation in order to combat persistent pulmonary hypertension (PPHN) and right-to-left shunting. The concept of gentle ventilation with permissive hypercapnea was pioneered by Charlie Stolar and Jen Wung's New York group during the 1990s, and intended to avoid barotraumatic lung injury in these fragile infants. Its roots lay the management of infants with persistent PPHN, where higher levels of $PaCO_2$ (50–60 mmHg) were accepted as a trade-off and the focus switched to preductal rather than postductal oxygen saturation levels as a measure of oxygen delivery (1). They then applied the same concepts to infants with CDH with some success, and reported its first use in the CDH infant in 1995 (2). Starting intermittent mandatory ventilation (IMV) settings were minimal: respiratory rate 40; inspiratory time 0.5; gas flow 5–7 L/min; peak inspiratory pressure (PIP) 20 cmH$_2$O; positive end-expiratory pressure (PEEP) 5 cmH$_2$O; and FiO$_2$ 1.0. PIP was adjusted according to chest excursion yet avoided the use of PIP > 25 cmH$_2$O, and infants were never hyperventilated to induce alkalisation. The FiO$_2$ rate was kept at minimum to maintain a pre-ductal saturation between 90–95%; however, a saturation level as low as 80% was accepted if the infant appeared comfortable and showing no signs of any organ dysfunction. Vigilant ventilation weaning strategy was adopted preoperatively, and FiO$_2$, ventilator rate and pressures were weaned as saturation and CO_2 clearance improved.

This is now considered the 'standard of care' in infants with CDH (3, 4).

REFERENCES

1. Wung JT, James LS, Kilchevsky E, James E. Management of infants with severe respiratory failure and persistence of the fetal circulation, without hyperventilation. Pediatrics. 1985;76(4):488–94.
2. Wung JT, Sahni R, Moffitt ST, Lipsitz E, Stolar CJ. Congenital diaphragmatic hernia: Survival treated with very delayed surgery, spontaneous respiration, and no chest tube. J Pediatr Surg. 1995;30(3):406–09.

3. Snoek KG, Reiss IKM, Greenough A, et al. Standardized postnatal management of infants with congenital diaphragmatic hernia in Europe: The CDH EURO Consortium Consensus – 2015 Update. Neonatology. 2016;110(1):66–74.

4. Ferguson DM, Gupta VS, Lally PA, et al. Early, postnatal pulmonary hypertension severity predicts inpatient outcomes in congenital diaphragmatic hernia. Neonatology. 2021;118(2):147–54.

CHAPTER 31

Extracorporeal Membrane Oxygenation (ECMO) for Newborn Respiratory Failure: 45 Cases

Bartlett RH, Andrews AF, Toomasian JM, Haiduc NJ, and Gazzaniga AB

Surgery 1982; 92:425–433.
Citations: *n* = 276

ABSTRACT

This paper described a Phase I trial of prolonged extracorporeal membrane oxygenation (ECMO) to provide life support while allowing the lung to 'rest' in 45 moribund newborn infants of which 25 survived.

The right atrium and aortic arch were cannulated via the jugular vein and carotid artery, and heparin was infused continuously to maintain an activated clotting time at 200 to 300 seconds. Airway oxygenation and pressure were reduced to low levels. The primary diagnoses were 'hyaline membrane disease' (respiratory distress syndrome) (*n* = 14, of which six survived); meconium aspiration syndrome (*n* = 22, of which 15 survived); persistent fetal circulation including diaphragmatic hernia (*n* = 5, of which three survived); and sepsis (*n* = 4, of which one survived).

Growth, development and brain and lung function were described as normal in 20 of 25 survivors.

COMMENTARY (MARK DAVENPORT)

The heart-lung machine was invented by John H Gibbon (1903–1973) and first used clinically in the early 1950s to replace heart and lung function long enough to allow operations on the heart. Its use in supporting cardiopulmonary function for longer periods was much more problematic, and success only occurred some decades later.

Robert (Bob) Bartlett (b. 1939) was the prime mover in the genesis of the American ECMO program. He started studying membrane oxygenators in the laboratories of Peter Bent Brigham Hospital, Boston, and Harvard Medical School with an engineer from the Massachusetts Institute of Technology (MIT), Phil Drinker. At that time, the aim was to support sick postoperative children who were recovering from cardiac surgery. Later, in 1975 and now in University of California, Irvine, with a fellow junior surgeon, Allan Gazzaniga, the team used ECMO for support of a newborn infant

DOI: 10.1201/9781003341901-31

with meconium aspiration and persistent fetal circulation. She was the daughter of an illegal immigrant from Mexico, but with the baby surviving the mother disappeared and the nurses named the baby Esperanza (Spanish for 'hope') as a summation of the crisis of the occasion (1).

This paper followed the relocation of the ECMO team to Ann Arbor, Michigan, and demonstrated the efficacy of the technique in a wide variety of conditions and scenarios.

The next step was to incorporate a randomized element to a trial design. This was called 'Play the Winner' and worked by randomizing the first case, then sticking to it if successful and reverting to the other if not. In the full-term infant arm, the first ECMO infant survived, and the next patient was a conventional treatment patient who died. The next ECMO patient survived, so the odds of being assigned to ECMO grew with each successive case. By the time 12 infants had been recruited, there were 11 in the ECMO group, all of whom survived, and one infant in the control group who had died.

The results were rejected by two journals before the third, *Pediatrics*, accepted it largely because of this unusual statistical trial format (2). There was another arm of the trial in preterm infants, but this was stopped early because of adverse events.

Later trials followed using more conventional randomization techniques (3), though still with relatively small numbers (e.g., $n = 39$, (4)). By 1990, virtually every major children's hospital in the USA had an ECMO team or a plan for triaging ECMO patients.

REFERENCES

1. Bartlett RH, Gazzaniga AB, Jefferies R, et al. Extracorporeal membrane oxygenation (ECMO) cardiopulmonary support in infancy. Trans Am Soc Artif Intern Organ. 1976;22:80–88.
2. Bartlett RH, Roloff DW, Cornell RG, et al. Extracorporeal circulation in neonatal respiratory failure: a prospective randomized study. Pediatrics. 1985;76:479–487.
3. Schumacher RE, Roloff DW, Chapman R, et al. Extracorporeal membrane oxygenation in term newborns: a prospective cost-benefit analysis. ASAIO J. 1993;39:873–879.
4. O'Rourke PP, Krone R, Vacanti J, et al. Extracorporeal membrane oxygenation and conventional medical therapy in neonates with persistent pulmonary hypertension of the newborn: a prospective randomized study. Pediatrics. 1989;84:957–963.

CHAPTER 32

Congenital Cystic Adenomatoid Malformation of the Lung. Classification and Morphologic Spectrum

Stocker JT, Madewell JE, and Drake RM

Human Pathology 1977 March; 8(2):155–171.
Citations: *n* = 834

ABSTRACT

'Thirty-eight cases of congenital cystic adenomatoid malformation (CCAM) of the lung are described, and a classification based on clinical, gross, and microscopic criteria is proposed ....'

The abstract then goes on to describe histological attributes of three types (Figure 32.1). Type I lesions (*n* = 19) being single or multiple large cysts (> 2 cm in diameter) lined by ciliated pseudostratified columnar epithelium. The walls of these cysts contain prominent smooth muscle, elastic tissue and mucus-producing cells.

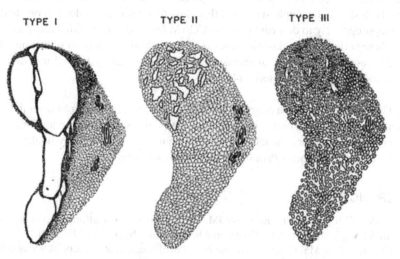

TYPE I   TYPE II   TYPE III

Figure 32.1 Stocker classification of CCAM. (Reproduced with permission.)

DOI: 10.1201/9781003341901-32

Type II lesions ($n = 16$) are composed of multiple small cysts (< 1 cm in diameter) lined by ciliated cuboidal to columnar epithelium. Type III lesions ($n = 3$) are large, bulky and noncystic. Bronchiole-like structures are lined by ciliated cuboidal epithelium.

The authors describe 38 cases taken from the (US) Armed Forces Institute of Pathology (AFIP) in Washington from as far back as 1917 to 1975. Clinical details of the infants and mothers were recorded. Ten patients had other abnormalities and typically renal agenesis. The outcomes for these patients were not given in any detail apart from suggesting that only Type I has any of sort of prognosis – with 11/16 surviving. All the rest died or were stillborn. This was a national reference laboratory, hence the large numbers in the series. As with most histological papers of this era, there are 19 black and white accompanying photographs.

COMMENTARY (MARK DAVENPORT)

An earlier paper was published in 1975 (1) in a radiology journal, this time with Madewell as the first author. The paper describes histology and X-ray features of 31 cases out of this AFIP series (and hence a lot of overlap!) but without any form of classification, which gives the latter paper its punch.

Up until this point, only something like 70 cases of CCAM had been published in the literature since its first acknowledged description in 1949, so this represents a huge part of existing knowledge to that point and quickly became definitive. The Stocker classification – Madewell and Drake were quickly airbrushed out – was modified in future years, not the least by Stocker himself and international consensus organisations (2). Two further types were recognized but rather than start the counting again, they were relabelled as Type 0 and Type IV to fit on either side. The whole was also submerged under the congenital pulmonary airways malformation (CPAM) umbrella. It should be emphasized that this classification is a histological one and is used inappropriately to describe possible CCAM lesions, particularly antenatally. For these, there is the Adzick classification (3), which is based simply on ultrasound (or magnetic resonance [MR]) characteristics and defines macrocystic (> 5 mm diameter) and microcystic (< 5 mm or solid) (4).

John Thomas Stocker was a major at the time of this paper and retired from the Armed Forces as a full colonel in 1995. He became the acknowledged authority on congenital respiratory pathology and wrote many classic pathology books (e.g., Stocker and Dehner's *Pediatric Pathology*) and papers.

REFERENCES

1. Madewell JE, Stocker JT, Korsower JM. Cystic adenomatoid malformation of the lung. Morphologic analysis. Am J Roentgenol Radium Ther Nucl Med. 1975;124(3):436–48.
2. Chin KY, Tang MY. Congenital adenomatoid malformation of one lobe of a lung with general anasarca. Arch Pathol. 1949;48:221.

3. Adzick NS, Harrison MR, Glick PL, Golbus MS, et al. Fetal cystic adenomatoid malformation: prenatal diagnosis and natural history. J Pediatr Surg. 1985;20(5):483–88.
4. Stocker JT. Congenital pulmonary airway malformation: a new name and expanded classification of congenital cystic adenomatoid malformation of the lung. Histopathology. 2002;41(2);424–31.

CHAPTER 33

Current Outcome of Antenatally Diagnosed Cystic Lung Disease

Mark Davenport, Stephanie A Warne, Sebastiano Cacciaguerra, Shailesh Patel, Anne Greenough, and Kypros Nicolaides

Journal of Pediatric Surgery 2004; 39(4):549–556.
Citations $n = 258$

ABSTRACT

This paper describes the outcomes of 67 fetuses with some kind of cystic lung abnormality antenatally diagnosed from January 1995 to July 2001. The Adzick classification was used, and these abnormalities were dominantly macrocystic ($n = 27$, 40%); microcystic ($n = 35$, 52%) and mixed ($n = 5$, 8%). A small number had had fetal intervention ($n = 4$, usually a thoracoamniotic shunt). Hydrops was present in five (7%). Sixty-four (96%) of the fetuses were born alive with one termination of pregnancy and two intrauterine deaths – all three having shown features of hydrops.

Open thoracotomy and excisional surgery was performed in 42 (63%) at a median of 7.5 months (range, one day to 34 months) with most being CCAM ($n = 25$), and the others pulmonary sequestrations ($n = 6$) or hybrid lesions ($n = 11$). There were two peri-operative deaths, both with severe disease and two air leaks requiring reinsertion of a chest tube before resolution. Twelve infants with small lesions were investigated but did not undergo surgery; rather, they were followed with serial imaging.

Some lesions appeared to have 'resolved' by the third trimester on ultrasound ($n = 10$), but imaging postnatally showed significant pathology in five, which were subsequently resected. Indeed, only two from the entire series on investigation seemed to have normal lungs.

Conclusion: antenatally diagnosed cystic lung disease (predominantly CCAM) has an excellent prognosis with an integrated approach to management.

COMMENTARY (MARK DAVENPORT)

Antenatal detection of significant pulmonary pathology was first described in the 1980s (1), and early series were bleak with reports of a high rate of associated major anomalies and *in utero* deaths, with poor survival overall (2, 3). Some physicians were even recommending elective terminations. This series was for a time the largest published single-centre experience of antenatally detected cystic lung lesions and

DOI: 10.1201/9781003341901-33

by contrast showed a much improved and more optimistic prognosis, with very favourable outcomes in the overwhelming majority. By advocating early surgery for those who were immediately symptomatic and thorough investigation using CT scan (not just X-rays) at about a month of life for even the asymptomatic subjects, a proper appreciation of the pathology could be undertaken.

This series was representative of a huge increase in numbers of infants with an antenatal diagnosis in newly established centres throughout the UK and Europe. In some UK centres, a more laissez-faire attitude to offering resection emerged for those deemed asymptomatic, which seemed anathema to American surgeons. This controversy has still to be resolved, although in the absence of randomisation this does not seem likely to happen in the near future (4, 5).

At the time, the Fetal Medicine Unit at King's College Hospital developed by Kypros Nicolaides, a pioneer in this new field, was the largest in Europe and worked closely with co-located surgeons and neonatal intensivists to provide a 'one-stop shop', a relative novelty at least in the UK. The increasing sensitivity and accuracy of antenatal ultrasound enabled better informed choices for prospective parents.

REFERENCES

1. Graham D, Winn K, Dex W, Sanders RC. Prenatal diagnosis of cystic adenomatoid malformation of the lung. J Ultrasound Med. 1982;1(1):9–12.
2. Kuller JA, Yankowitz J, Goldberg JD, Harrison MR, et al. Outcome of antenatally diagnosed cystic adenomatoid malformations. Am J Obstet Gynecol. 1992;167(4 Pt 1):1038–41.
3. Thorpe-Beeston JG, Nicolaides KH. Cystic adenomatoid malformation of the lung: prenatal diagnosis and outcome. Prenat Diagn. 1994;14(8):677–88.
4. Singh R, Davenport M. The argument for operative approach to asymptomatic lung lesions. Semin Pediatr Surg. 2015;24(4):187–95.
5. Stanton M. The argument for a non-operative approach to asymptomatic lung lesions. Semin Pediatr Surg. 2015;24(4):183–86.

CHAPTER 34

A 10-Year Review of a Minimally Invasive Technique for the Correction of Pectus Excavatum

Donald Nuss, Robert E Kelly Jr, Daniel P Croitoru, and Michael E Katz

Journal of Pediatric Surgery 1998; 33(4):545–552
Citations: *n* = 991

ABSTRACT

This was a report from the Children's Hospital of the King's Daughters, Norfolk, Virginia, on the tenth anniversary of the Nuss procedure, a minimally invasive approach in the management of pectus excavatum.

This was a retrospective single-centre series of children < 15 years presenting between 1987 and 1996.

Those with pectus excavatum underwent an initial physiotherapy and posture program, and correction was offered for those who failed this conservative approach. CT thorax was performed preoperatively in the last 12 cases. Haller's index was calculated by dividing the transverse chest diameter by the anteroposterior diameter. Patients were photographed before and after surgery, and the response to surgery was graded: excellent, normal chest; good, mild residual pectus; fair, moderate residual pectus; and poor, severe recurrence requiring further treatment.

The Nuss technique involved creating a retrosternal tunnel between two thoracic incisions using a curved Kelly clamp and then placing a 1.5 cm wide and 2 mm thick steel bar (initially titanium was used) to lift the sternum forward. The steel bar was inserted with the convex edge facing posteriorly, and once in position the bar was turned 180°, raising the sternum and anterior chest wall to the desired position. A second bar above or below was also placed if it was thought necessary. The bar was secured with heavy sutures to the lateral chest wall muscles. In the first three years, the Nuss technique included an anterior thoracic incision to aid bar insertion, while after 1991 only lateral incisions were used.

Patients were discharged from the hospital when able to walk unaided. Regular activity was permitted whenever the patient was fully recovered, usually at the end of 30 days. The bars were left for a minimum of two years.

DOI: 10.1201/9781003341901-34

Results: One hundred forty-eight children presented with a chest wall deformity (pectus excavatum, $n = 127$, mostly boys, $n = 104$). Of those, 50/127 (39%) underwent surgery, the Ravitch procedure ($n = 8$) and the new Nuss approach ($n = 42$). The age at the time of the Nuss procedure ranged between 15 months and 15 years but was mainly (21/50) in the four to five years age group. The main presenting symptom in the surgery group was exercise intolerance and exertional dyspnoea (16/50) followed by recurrent upper respiratory chest infections (15/50). Twelve patients had a CT thorax preoperatively, and the median (range) Haller index was 5.5 (3.1–8.5). Mean LOS was 4.3 (three to seven) days.

Postoperative complications occurred in 12/42 (28%), and three (7%) required further surgical intervention. Pneumothorax occurred in four patients (10%); three were unilateral, in the immediate postoperative period and resolved spontaneously within 24 hours. The last was bilateral pneumothorax in a 15-year-old trumpet player two months after surgery and required chest drain placement. Bar repositioning was required in two cases due to insufficient initial stabilisation. Recurrence of excavatum anomaly requiring further corrective surgery was reported in three cases (7%) after the Nuss procedure.

The mean follow-up time was 4.6 (1–9.2) years, and the mean follow-up from bar removal (in 30/42) was 2.8 years (6 months – 7). The one-year postbar removal response was graded: excellent in 22 patients, good in four and fair or poor in another four.

Conclusion: The Nuss procedure provides a minimally invasive alternative in pectus excavatum repair with very good cosmetic outcomes.

COMMENTARY (BASHAR ALDEIRI)

Donald Nuss is a South African surgeon working in a relatively small and quaintly named children's hospital in Norfolk, Virginia. He performed his first case in 1986 following the observation that the costal cartilages in the younger child were relatively malleable and could be elevated and supported by a metal bar inserted underneath without actual resection. This surgical principle underlies the Nuss procedure and modifications that followed and provided a practical, relatively minimally invasive alternative to the operations that preceded it. Typically, this had been the Ravitch procedure, which required a long anterior chest incision and fracturing and resetting of the costal cartilages (1).

The procedure gained wide acceptance and a lot of referrals. A literature review in 2008 identified almost 2,000 published cases (2) without any mortality, and a follow-up series from the original center in Virginia published in the 2010 *Annals of Surgery* could report the experience of 1,215 cases (3).

While the procedure was offered initially to younger prepubertal children with pectus excavatum, it is now typically deferred until their teenage years (4). The change of bar material to stainless steel has already been mentioned, titanium being too soft. The split between one or two bars is about 50:50 (4). Bilateral thoracoscopy was also introduced in 1998, allowing direct visualisation (appealing to the safety conscious) during the substernal dissection. Sternal elevation also seemed to improve the safety of the substernal dissection, and a variety of retractors and suction cups have been developed. The use of stabilizer bars since 1998 reduced the incidence of bar displacement, and in 2002 the addition of pericostal suture reduced the rate of bar displacement to < 1% (4). Preoperative allergy testing to stainless steel (~10%) may also avoid some of the immune-related issues. Much of the latest work seems to be to try to get these children and young people out of hospital faster, acknowledging that it is a painful procedure with the use of nerve blocks and cryoablation (5).

REFERENCES

1. Ravitch MM. The operative treatment of pectus excavatum. Ann Surg. 1949;129:429–44.
2. Protopapas AD, Athanasiou T. Peri-operative data on the Nuss procedure in children with pectus excavatum: independent survey of the first 20 years' data. J Cardiothorac Surg. 2008;3:40.
3. Kelly RE, Goretsky MJ, Obermeyer R, Kuhn MA, et al. Twenty-one years of experience with minimally invasive repair of pectus excavatum by the Nuss procedure in 1215 patients. Ann Surg. 2010;252:1072–81.
4. Kelly RE Jr, Obermeyer RJ, Goretsky MJ, Kuhn MA, et al. Recent modifications of the nuss procedure: the pursuit of safety during the minimally invasive repair of pectus excavatum. Ann Surg. 2022;275(2):e496–e502.
5. Graves CE, Moyer J, Zobel MJ, Mora R, et al. Intraoperative intercostal nerve cryoablation during the Nuss procedure reduces length of stay and opioid requirement: a randomized clinical trial. J Pediatr Surg. 2019;54:2250–56.

CHAPTER 35

Vincristine Sulphate and Cyclophosphamide for Children with Metastatic Neuroblastoma

Audrey E Evans, Ruth M Heyns, William A Newton Jr, and Sanford L Leikin

Journal of the American Medical Association 1969 February 17; 207(7):1325–1327.
Citations: $n = 34$

ABSTRACT

Thirty-eight children with metastatic neuroblastoma were given a combination of vincristine sulphate and cyclophosphamide in addition to standard surgical and radiotherapeutic management. The two agents were given intravenously on alternating weeks for 12 weeks or longer.Results were best in eight infants under one year, five of whom continued to survive free of disease for 16 months. The overall response rate in patients of all ages was 32% (nine out of 28), and the mean survival was 12 months.

The combination of the two agents was effective.

COMMENTARY (MARK DAVENPORT)

Neuroblastoma (NB) is the most common extracranial solid tumour in children, with rates of metastases at diagnosis of 60–70%. This American multi-institutional study sought to tackle what is still a very difficult and potentially fatal disease – high-risk NB. Enthusiasm for drug therapy increased after James et al. in 1965 reported five survivors from nine consecutive unresectable neuroblastomas (1).

Both of the chemotherapeutic agents used here had shown a degree of effectiveness when used in isolation previously, and this paper suggested improvement when combined. Objective regression was seen in about a 1/3 with obvious improvement in infants, where about 50% were in complete remission.

Since the 1960s, there has been increasing use of a variety of toxic chemotherapy strategies to try to achieve and then sustain remission in high-risk NB. Current treatment for high-risk NB can be divided into three distinct phases: induction of remission, consolidation of the remission and finally a maintenance phase focused on the eradication of minimal residual disease. It is dogmatic that increasing the intensity of induction chemotherapy is associated with improvements in response rates and overall survival rates (2). Deliberate bone marrow ablation and stem cell rescue was introduced during the 1990s to try to raise this particular ceiling, and that does seem to have improved event-free survival, although the effect on overall survival still seems to be contentious (3). Surprisingly, more than 50 years later, both chemotherapy agents used here retain a place in the current armamentarium with additional agents, including cisplatin, etoposide and doxorubicin.

Surgeons still have a role in high-risk NB. Resection should follow an induction chemotherapy regimen. The effects of the degree of that resection are also debated. Systematic analysis has shown that there is no difference in the five-year event-free survival or overall survival between complete surgical resection or gross tumour resection (4). So what does this all mean today? Well, unfortunately, estimated long-term survival for high-risk NB is still only about 40–50%.

The first author on this paper was the remarkable Audrey Elizabeth Evans (1925–2022), born in England but working predominantly after qualification in the USA, where she was known as the "Mother of Neuroblastoma". She had been tasked by 'Chick' Everitt Koop in 1968 with setting up the first paediatric oncology unit at the Children's Hospital of Philadelphia. Here she invented the Evans classification (5), one of the first prognostic classifications for NB, and also first described spontaneous regression in some cases of what was later termed Stage IVS disease (6).

REFERENCES

1. James DH Jr, Hustu O, Wrenn EL. Combination chemotherapy of childhood neuroblastoma, JAMA. 1965;194:123–126.
2. Maris JM. Recent advances in neuroblastoma. N Engl J Med. 2010;362(23):2202–2211.
3. Yalçin B, Kremer LCM, Caron HN, van Dalen EC. High-dose chemotherapy and autologous haematopoietic stem cell rescue for children with high-risk neuroblastoma. Cochrane Database Syst Rev. 2013;22(8):CD006301. doi: 10.1002/14651858.CD006301. pub3
4. Qi Y, Zhan J. Roles of surgery in the treatment of patients with high-risk neuroblastoma in the children oncology group study: A systematic review and meta-analysis. Front Pediatr. 2021;9:706800. doi: 10.3389/fped.2021.706800
5. Evans AE, D'Angio GJ, Judson R. A proposed staging for children with neuroblastoma. Cancer. 1971;27:374–378.
6. Evans AE, Baum E, Chard R. Do infants with stage IV-S neuroblastoma need treatment? Arch Dis Child. 1981;56:271–274.

CHAPTER 36

The Treatment of Wilms' Tumor. Results of the National Wilms' Tumor Study

D'Angio GJ, Evans AE, Breslow N, Beckwith B, Bishop H, Feigl P, Goodwin W, Leape LL, Sinks LF, Sutow W, Tefft M, and Wolff J

Cancer 1976; 38(2):633–646.
Citations: $n = 365$

ABSTRACT

The National Wilms' Tumor Study (NWTS), initiated in 1969, tested competing treatment strategems for patients with tumours ranging from Group (Gp) I (tumours confined to the kidney and totally removed) to Gp IV (remote metastases present at diagnosis).

Three hundred fifty-nine of 606 registered patients were randomized in the trial.

- Gp I patients < 2 years of age fared well whether postoperative radiation therapy (RT) was or was not added to 15 months' maintenance actinomycin D (AMD). Their prognosis was better than that for older cohorts similarly treated, in whom the difference in relapse rates between treatment groups were suggestive of an RT effect.
- Combined AMD and vincristine (VCR) gave better results than either agent alone in patients with more advanced tumours (Gps II and III) still confined to the abdomen. All of these patients received postoperative RT as well (Figure 36.1).
- Preoperative VCR given to Gp IV patients in addition to postoperative RT, AMD and VCR did not improve results.

The frequency of mesoblastic nephroma (1%), of bilateral tumours (5%), and of incorrect preoperative diagnosis of Wilms' tumor (5%), the toxicities of the various regimens and other ancillary data are presented and discussed.

DOI: 10.1201/9781003341901-36

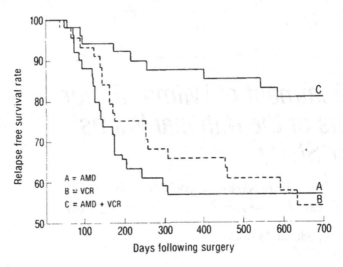

Figure 36.1   Relapse-free survival in Gp II and III (A vs B vs C).

COMMENTARY (BASHAR ALDEIRI)

The evolution of the multimodal modern management of Wilms' tumor is one of the success stories of contemporary paediatric surgery, and due credit is rightly given to the American NWTS and Societe Internationale D'oncologie Pediatrique (SIOP), its European equivalent, in designing and carrying out big clinical trials. Nevertheless, as Wilms' tumors are heterogenous in terms of stage, biology and response to treatment, such treatment arms are complex and the results sometimes difficult to tease out.

One of the first landmarks in Wilms' management was the introduction of the antibiotic Actinomycin D into oncology by Sidney Farber (1903–1973) in the Boston Children's Hospital in 1960 (1). The synergetic effect of this new chemotherapeutic agent alongside radiotherapy achieved a dramatic improvement in the two-year survival rate reaching the 80% figure for the first time in the history of management of this tumour. However, the paucity of cases made it hard for any single institution to have the volume of cases to test these emerging treatments individually or in combination and validate their superiority in an objective clinical trial assessment. This led to the formation of the National Wilms' Tumor Study Group in 1968, led by Giulio D'Angio, a radiotherapist from the Children's Hospital of Philadelphia. D'Angio recruited surgeons, oncologists and radiotherapists with clear set of objectives to develop and refine treatment protocols and study the natural history of Wilms' tumor, with an overriding goal that 'cure is not enough' when addressing children with cancer (2, 3).

Figure 36.2 illustrates the allocated treatment web for this, the 1st NWTS co-operative study. The primary end point of the study was relapse-free survival. This study

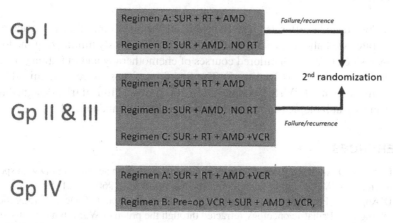

Figure 36.2 Treatment allocation NWTS.

randomized 359 of the 606 cases registered in the NWTS (Gp I, n = 163; GpII, n = 100; Gp III, n = 100; and Gp IV, n = 26).

Group I NWTS

Age stratification showed that children (< 24 months) had a very good prognosis ± radiotherapy. The overall relapse-free survival rate after two years of follow-up was 67% in comparison to 89% (< 2 years, P = 0.002). In the > 2-year group, relapse-free survival rates in the radiated and nonradiated groups were 77% and 58% respectively (P = 0.04). The overall survival in Group I was comparable between the two treatment regimens in all age groups and in the two age subgroups (< 2 years and ≥ 2 years).

Groups II–III NWTS

The use of combination therapy (AMD and VCR) yielded a better survival and disease-free survival in patients with regional spread of the disease (Figure 36.1) (80% in the combined therapy group vs 55% in the VCR alone). The outcome of the AMD alone varied according to the disease stage with an overall survival of 72% in Group II patients as oppose to 44% in Group III.

Groups IV NWTS

In the 26 cases that were randomized there were 2/13 deaths in the immediate surgery group as opposed to 9/13 in the preoperative VCR group (P = 0.2).

Treatment Toxicity

The treatment was well tolerated in all age groups. However, there were ten treatment-related (toxicity or infection) mortalities amongst the 359 children treated (3%).

Six of these deaths were in children receiving intense treatment after a relapse of the primary tumour.

Just over two decades after its birth, the National Wilms' Tumor Study had achieved survival rates well above the 95% mark, while simultaneously minimizing the long-term toxic side effects with tailored courses of chemotherapy and radiation (3). NWTS ran five clinical trials (NWTS-1 to -5). The first four of these were randomized trials, whereas the last one (NWTS-5 completed in 2003) was a clinical trial designed to look primarily at biologic prognostic factors and was not randomized.

REFERENCES

1. Farber S, D'Angio G, Evans A, Mitus A. Clinical studies on actinomycin D with special reference to Wilms' tumor in children. Ann NY Acad Sci. 1960;89:421–5.
2. D'Angio GJ. Pediatric cancer in perspective: cure is not enough. Cancer. 1975;35:866–70.
3. D'Angio G. Pediatric oncology refracted through the prism of Wilms tumor: a discourse. J Urol. 2000;164:2073–7.

CHAPTER 37

Effectiveness and Toxicity of Cisplatin and Doxorubicin (PLADO) in Childhood Hepatoblastoma and Hepatocellular Carcinoma: A SIOP Pilot Study

Jacques Ninane, Giorgio Perilongo, Jean-Phillipe Stalens, Maurizio Guglielmi, Jean-Bernard Otte, and Antonia Mancini

Medical and Pediatric Oncology. 1991; 19:199–203.
Citations: $n = 73$

ABSTRACT

This was a pilot study by the European paediatric oncology organisation Societe Internationale D'oncologie Pediatrique (SIOP), using the novel chemotherapy regime PLADO (*plat*inum *dox*orubicin) in paediatric liver tumours.

Methods: Children with histological confirmation of epithelial liver tumours diagnosed consecutively between June 1987 and October 1989 were treated in five European centres (Brussels, Belgium and four Italian centres within the Italian Liver Tumour Study Group).

PLADO consisted of a three-day continuous infusion regime of Cisplatin (CDDP) and doxorubicin (DOXO). On day 1, children received CDDP CI; in Brussels, this was given at a dose of 80 mg/m2 IV over 24 hours, and in Italy at a dose of 90 mg/m^2 over six hours. Days 2 and 3 consisted of DOXO infusion over 48 hours at a dose of 60 mg/m^2. The PLADO course was repeated at three weekly intervals.

After four cycles of PLADO, tumour response and surgical resectability were evaluated by repeating computed tomography (CT) scans of the lungs and liver. Complete response (CR) was defined as complete resolution of all evidence of tumour, very good partial response (VGPR) as > 75% reduction in tumour volume, partial response (PR) as any lesser tumour size shrinkage and stable disease (SD) as the lack of any tumour volume reduction. Following complete tumour resection, patients received either two further PLADO courses or no further therapy.

Toxicity was assessed after each course of chemotherapy and graded according to the World Health Organisation (WHO) toxicity grading system. Cardiac toxicity was monitored by repeated electrocardiograms (ECG) and echocardiograms, renal toxicity by renal function tests and hepatic toxicity by liver transaminases levels. All children underwent an audiogram hearing assessment.

Results: Sixteen children were treated (hepatoblastoma [HB], $n = 13$ and hepatocellular carcinoma [HCC], $n = 3$). The median age at diagnosis was two (16 days – 13) years. Extrahepatic (pulmonary) disease was present only in one case of HB, while all other tumours were confined to the liver.

Ten patients received preoperative chemotherapy, nine of which were HB. The number of PLADO cycles was two in one case, three in one case and four in the remaining eight. The response to treatment was VGPR ($n = 7$), PR ($n = 2$) (50% and 35%), and no response in one HB case. The first nine cases underwent complete resection of the primary tumour, while the no-responder underwent a liver transplant. Seven patients received postoperative chemotherapy; five received two courses, and two received four. All patients were alive with no signs of recurrence after a median follow-up of 12 (4–32) months.

Six children had primary surgery, four of which received four courses of PLADO postoperatively. One later developed pulmonary metastasis, while the rest are alive with no signs of residual disease. Two cases of HB in this group were initially followed up postoperatively without planned chemotherapy. Both developed pulmonary metastasis and has subsequently received delayed chemotherapy (eight and ten PLADO cycles), and both showed complete response and were alive at the time of the last follow-up.

The toxicity of the new PLADO regime was assessed in all cases using the WHO grading system, where Grade 2 or more is considered severe toxicity. All 16 patients showed signs of severe myelosuppression, and 11 developed an infection requiring intravenous antibiotics, five of which were central line infections. One HB patient in the primary surgery group, who subsequently received ten cycles of PLADO, developed CDDP-acquired hearing loss and DOXO-associated cardiomyopathy. None of the 16 patients developed a Grade 2 or higher renal or hepatic toxicity.

Conclusion: PLADO appears to be an effective regime to induce response in childhood hepatocellular malignancy with an acceptable level of toxicity.

COMMENTARY (BASHAR ALDEIRI)

Hepatoblastoma was almost invariably fatal prior to the introduction of neoadjuvant chemotherapy. In the largest published cohort of childhood hepatic tumours from a survey of North America centres in the 1970s, Exelby et al. (1) reported an overall survival rate in HB in 35%. This ranged from 60%, where complete resection was feasible, to none, when partial resection of the tumour was attempted.

The introduction of combined chemotherapy regimens in the 1970s to shrink the tumour and treat distal seeding was shown to improve disease-free survival and overall survival in children with hepatic tumours (2). The introduction of cisplatin- and doxorubicin-containing regimens in the 1980s had a major impact on overall survival. This SIOP pilot study was the first milestone in the modern approach in the management of HB. It also standardised the use of biopsy to confirm the diagnosis, introduced the concept of neoadjuvant chemotherapy and alluded to a risk stratification strategy. It led the way to the first study by the liver group of the International Society of Pediatric Oncology (SIOPEL 1 study) that proved the value of preoperative (PLADO) chemotherapy, leading to a staggering five-year survival of 75% and event-free survival of 66% (3).

The management of hepatoblastoma has evolved over the last 30 years, yet PLADO remains the backbone of the chemotherapy regimen.

REFERENCES

1. Exelby PR, Filler RM, Grosfeld JL. Liver tumors in children in the particular reference to hepatoblastoma and hepatocellular carcinoma: American Academy of Pediatrics Surgical Section Survey-1974. J Pediatr Surg. 1975;10:329–37.
2. Evans AE, Land VJ, Newton WA, et al. Combination chemotherapy (vincristine, adriamycin, cyclophosphamide, and 5-fluorouracil) in the treatment of children with malignant hepatoma. Cancer. 1982;50:821–26.
3. Pritchard J, Brown J, Shafford E, et al. Cisplatin, doxorubicin, and delayed surgery for childhood hepatoblastoma: A successful approach–results of the first prospective study of the International Society of Pediatric Oncology. J Clin Oncol. 2000;18(22):3819–28.

CHAPTER 38

Correction of Experimentally Produced Vesicoureteric Reflux in the Piglet by Intravesical Injection of Teflon

Prem Puri and Barry O'Donnell

British Medical Journal 1984; 289(6436):5–7.
Citations: *n* = 135

Treatment of Vesicoureteric Reflux by Endoscopic Injection of Teflon

Barry O'Donnell and Prem Puri

British Medical Journal 1984; 289(6436):7–9.
Citations: *n* = 338

ABSTRACT (HUMAN STUDY)

'Thirteen girls with grade III-V vesicoureteric reflux were treated by endoscopic injection of Teflon paste behind the intravesical ureter. Fourteen of the 18 treated ureters showed complete absence of reflux after one injection of Teflon. Three ureters required a second injection of Teflon for successful treatment of the reflux. One ureter with grade IV reflux was converted to grade H reflux. Properly carried out, this procedure corrects reflux. It takes less than 15 minutes, may be done as a day procedure, and avoids open surgery. There have been no complications.'

... 'We call the procedure "The Sting" – that is, Subureteric Teflon **Ing**ection.'

COMMENTARY (PREM PURI)

My interest in vesicoureteral reflux (VUR) started in the late 1970s when I was working as a research fellow with Professor Barry O'Donnell in Dublin. In the 1970s and 1980s, there was general agreement that children with higher grades of VUR and those with breakthrough urinary tract infections should have antireflux surgery. I saw one or two ureteral reimplantation procedures being done every week in my hospital. I felt that reimplantation of ureters was too major a procedure just to anchor the intravesical ureter to the bladder. I said to Professor O'Donnell that it should

                                    DOI: 10.1201/9781003341901-38

be possible to inject a bulking agent endoscopically behind the submucosal ureter that would not only give a solid support but also provide a firm anchorage for the intravesical ureter. Professor O'Donnell said to me 'great idea'. I wrote a research grant application in 1982 and induced VUR in two- to four-week-old piglets by opening the bladder and slitting the anterior wall of both intravesical ureters and cured VUR by injecting Teflon paste subureterically. The experimental correction allowed us to begin treating patients with VUR endoscopically in March 1984. We published two papers in the *British Medical Journal* on July 7, 1984. The first paper was on correction of experimentally produced VUR in the piglet, and the second paper was on the treatment of VUR in 13 girls by endoscopic subureteral injection of Teflon. Fourteen of the 18 treated ureters with grade III-V VUR showed complete absence of reflux after a single endoscopic injection of Teflon paste.

Our two articles in the *British Medical Journal* generated lot of interest amongst pediatric urologists, pediatric surgeons and pediatric nephrologists worldwide, and they started treating VUR by the 15-minute day care endoscopic procedure. However, in 1991, Ian Aaronson, a pediatric urologist from South Carolina, reported distant particle migration following intravesical injection of Teflon in dogs (1). Following this report, we conducted very detailed studies in dogs and minipigs and reported in 1994 that there was no distant particle migration following subureteral injection of Teflon on histological examination, polarised light microscopy, scanning electron microscopy and X-ray microanalysis. Several other bulking agents were now being used endoscopically to treat VUR, including collagen, autologous fat, polydimethylsiloxane, silicone, chondrocytes and dextranomer/hyaluronic acid (Dx/HA or Deflux™)

The greatest paradigm shift in the endoscopic treatment of VUR occurred when the American regulator, the Food and Drug Administration (FDA), approved Deflux™ as an acceptable tissue-augmenting substance for the endoscopic treatment of VUR in children in 2001. Another important milestone in the endoscopic treatment of VUR was in 2002. This year, the *Journal of Urology* accorded "Classic Article Status" to a few important urological articles published in the last century which had major impact on patient treatment worldwide. Our article published in the *British Medical Journal* in 1984 was accorded "Classic Article" status. Now there was a worldwide acceptance that Deflux™ is an effective and safe tissue-augmenting substance in the endoscopic treatment of VUR. It is estimated that over a million children with VUR have been treated worldwide endoscopically since publication in 1984.

COMMENTARY (BASHAR ALDEIRI)

This was Prem Puri and Barry O'Donnell's first report from Our Lady's Hospital for Sick Children, Crumlin, Dublin, describing what became known as the "STING" procedure standing for, somewhat imaginatively, Subureteric Teflon INGection.

The sister paper published in the same issue of the *British Medical Journal* with the order of the authors' names reversed described the preliminary porcine model of VUR treated with intravesical Teflon injection. Artificial VUR was created surgically in eight piglets, and the presence of VUR was confirmed on micturating cystogram (MCUG). After six to eight weeks the animals were treated with an intravesical injection of Teflon. At the last study time point, at six months, all animals had complete resolution of VUR and no signs of mechanical obstruction at the vesicoureteric junction (VUJ) was noted after a single injection of Teflon.

The treatment of VUR in children was controversial then as it is today, but open surgical procedures were very much in vogue, particularly the Cohen reimplantation (2). This endoscopic alternative by comparison was minimally invasive and appeared as effective.

The first report of endoscopic treatment of VUR using intravesical Teflon injection was by Matouschek in the Spanish Archives of Urology in 1981 (3). The choice to use Teflon (or polytetrafluoroethylene) at the time was not random. The material was widely used by urologists treating adults in the 1960s and 1970s as a bulking agent around the urethra to manage urinary incontinence. The STING replicated the concepts behind ureteric reimplantation without the need of invasive surgery and created a longer intravesical ureter. Standard cystourethroscopy using a 14F scope was performed and the bladder was filled with saline. A specially designed 5Fg polyethylene catheter ending in an 18-gauge needle was used. The needle was inserted 2–3 mm caudal to the ureteric orifice and advanced into the space behind it. Then 0.2–0.5 ml Polytef™ paste (Ethicon) was injected into this subureteric space.

There was an enthusiastic uptake of the new approach, at least in Europe, with many convincing reports of excellent long-term outcomes. Nowadays, while the STING as a procedure continues, the use of Teflon as an injectable material has been nearly abandoned. Teflon was stiff and difficult to inject, and there were concerning reports regarding the possibility of particle migration to the lungs and brain (1). Other materials took its place with the current favourite being dextranomer/hyaluronic acid (Dx/HA, Deflux™, Salix Pharmaceuticals, NJ, USA) (4).

Modifications to the actual technique of injection also occurred, and even more acronyms were invented. So, another current favourite is the HIT, or even the double HIT (for hydrodistention implantation technique) (5). This needle is introduced into the submucosa inside the ureteral tunnel to achieve a better co-aption of the wall of the ureter.

REFERENCES

1. Aaronson IA, Rames RA, Greene WB, Walsh LG, Hasal UA, Garen PD. Endoscopic treatment of reflux: migration of Teflon to the lungs and brain. Eur Urol. 1993;23(3):394–9.
2. Cohen SJ. Ureterozystoneostomie: eine neue antireflux Technik. Aktuel Urol. 1975;6:1–9.
3. Matouschek E. [New concept for the treatment of vesico-ureteral reflux. Endoscopic application of teflon]. Arch Esp Urol. 1981;34(5):385–8.

4. Escolino M, Kalfa N, Castagnetti M, Caione P, et al. Endoscopic injection of bulking agents in pediatric vesicoureteral reflux: a narrative review of the literature. Pediatr Surg Int. 2023;39(1):133. doi: 10.1007/s00383-023-05426-w

5. Kirsch AJ, Perez-Brayfield M, Smith EA, Scherz HC. The modified Sting procedure to correct vesicoureteral reflux: improved results with submucosal implantation within the intra mural ureter. J Urol. 2004;171(6 Pt 1):2413–6.

CHAPTER 39

Preliminary Report
The Antegrade Continence Enema

Padraig S Malone, Philip G Ransley, Edward M Kiely

Lancet 1990; 336(8725):1217–1218.
Citations: *n* = 700

ABSTRACT

'The principles of antegrade colonic washout and the Mitrofanoff non-refluxing catheterisable channel were combined to produce a continent catheterisable colonic stoma. The intention was that antegrade washouts delivered by this route would produce complete colonic emptying and thereby prevent soiling. The procedure has been successfully carried out in five patients with intractable faecal incontinence (Figure 39.1).'

COMMENTARY (BASHAR ALDEIRI)

This report from Great Ormond Street Hospital, London proposed a novel method of clearing the colon and provided the community with another acronym – the antegrade continent enema (ACE), or later, the Malone antegrade continent enema (MACE) procedure if you prefer.

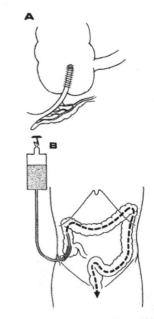

Non-refluxing appendicocaecostomy (A) and ACE principle (B).

Figure 39.1 Nonrefluxing appendicocaecostomy (A) and ACE principle (B). (Courtesy of Elsevier.)

Five girls, aged between eight and 18 years, with intractable faecal incontinence, had their appendix reimplanted between the caecum and the skin to create a nonrefluxing catheterisable channel that allowed performing antegrade colonic washout. Of these, three with myelomeningocele and one with a cloacal anomaly had the procedure as part of a concurrent bladder reconstructive procedure to address urinary incontinence. One girl with an anorectal malformation had it performed in isolation.

DOI: 10.1201/9781003341901-39

Essentially, the appendix with a cuff of the caecum was mobilised and detached from the rest of the caecum while preserving its blood supply. It was then reversed and the distal end of the appendix implanted into a submucosal caecal tunnel to create a nonrefluxing channel. The proximal end was anchored to a skin-flap tube in the lower abdomen. A catheter was left in the new channel for two to three weeks to allow healing, and antegrade colonic washouts started from day ten. The new channel was accessed every two to three days to deliver a 'bespoke' washout regime that consisted of sodium phosphate and isotonic saline solution. Four of the five patients needed to perform a washout every 48 hours, while one managed with every 72 hours. All patients used sodium phosphate in the washout solution, and four used an extra volume of sodium chloride ranged between 80 and 400 mls. The maximum time taken to deliver the washout ranged between 20–30 minutes. All patients reported improved faecal continence with the new approach. Two patients reported leakage of washout fluid, and one patient had a skin-level stomal stenosis. The follow-up period ranged between two to eight months.

Management of faecal incontinence in neuropathic bowel and high anorectal malformation at the time was challenging, and most cases eventually required a permanent stoma. One of the early successful reports in achieving 'social faecal continence' came from Shandling and Gilmour from the Sick Kids Hospital, Toronto, in 1987 (1). They reported the use of colonic irrigation via a rectal catheter in over 100 children and adolescents with neuropathic bowel and managed to achieve satisfactory faecal continence. This concept revolutionised the management of neuropathic bowel and gained favour amongst clinicians and surgeons at the time. Similarly, the Mitrofanoff concept of creating a nonrefluxing catheterisable channel to achieve urinary continence started to become popular following John Duckett's and Howard Snyder's series in 1986 (2). Padraig Malone combined the two concepts to allow the delivery of colonic washout in an antegrade fashion through a catheterisable channel accessed from the abdomen in order to deliver it. The former ensured better clearance of the colon, while the latter promoted autonomy and independence and avoided reliance on accessing the anus in the many 'wheelchair-user' patients.

MACE emerged from what Malone described as 'frustration'. In his years of training, Pat Malone worked for Philip Ransley, a paediatric urologist at Great Ormond Street Hospital. Pat used to feel frustrated when patients, following a major urinary reconstruction delivering continence, came back to their clinic still wearing nappies, i.e., they were still *faecally* incontinent. While they had succeeded in protecting the renal tract and achieving urinary continence, they actually made very little difference to the patient and the family's quality of life overall. The frustration that he had not been able to make a lasting difference was the drive that guided Malone in his search. He then recalled a technique from his general surgery training in Worcester Royal Infirmary, where they used to perform on-table antegrade colonic irrigation by catheterising the appendix and flushing the colon clear prior to performing primary colonic anastomosis. The penny then dropped and Malone came up with the idea of creating a Mitrofanoff for the caecum. It all made total sense. This would allow intermittent catheterisation of the colon, delivering an antegrade washout that will clear the colon, resulting in continence for a couple of days, which can then repeated. There was only one little hurdle to overcome: he needed to sell the idea to his boss at the time, Philip Ransley. What could beat a pint in a pub on a Friday evening after a long operating list to introduce his big idea. Reportedly, the response was, 'That is the most stupid idea I have ever heard in all my life'. Nevertheless, it did not take Ransley long to see the potential of Malone's novel idea, and by Monday morning he had signed up, and within a few months, together with the paediatric surgeon Edward Kiely, trialled the technique in six patients as described.

The MACE procedure gained wide acceptance and was instantly embraced by paediatric and adult surgeons (3). A plethora of modifications was proposed in the next decade, but they all kept the appendix attached to the caecum proximally and used various imbrication methods to create a nonrefluxing appendix conduit. However, it soon became evident that the mainstay of the technique was simply to create a catheterisable channel. Reimplanting the appendix in a submucosal caecal tunnel, a concept derived from the urinary principle of creating an antireflux tunnel in ureteroneocystostomy, was somewhat redundant. The risk of significant retrograde faecal leakage through the conduit is low given that the colon is a 'low-pressure system' and essentially harmless. In 2000, Savage and Yohannes introduced a simplified version of the MACE that they performed laparoscopically (4). They simply brought the distal end of the appendix out through a 5 mm port site in the right iliac fossa and created a stoma, while the appendix was still attached to the caecum proximally. The appendix was accessed with a relatively small-sized tube (5–8 Fg) in order to deliver washout, and the authors achieved good continence control and did not encounter any significant retrograde leakage. This is probably the most widely practised variant nowadays, and has largely replaced all other historic techniques.

The long-term fate of the ACE is still a matter of debate. Long-term follow-up studies demonstrated that the approach, at first, is effective in childhood and young adults with good faecal continence control. However, these reports suggest that ACE management generally becomes less optimal over time. In one study, a third of the patients have stopped accessing the ACE after a decade, and this was mainly due to poor results (5). Many patients in adulthood find managing a stoma preferable to continue with their MACE washouts.

Thirty years on, the MACE procedure remains a pillar of modern bowel management protocols.

I would like to thank Mr Padraig Malone for allowing me to use some of the comments and events he listed in his recent podcast *Circumsession* in the writing of this chapter (6).

REFERENCES

1. Shandling B, Gilmour RF. The enema continence catheter in spina bifida: successful bowel management. J Pediatr Surg. 1987;22(3):271–3.
2. Duckett JW, Snyder HM 3rd. Continent urinary diversion: variations on the Mitrofanoff principle. J Urol. 1986;136:58–62.
3. Curry JI, Osborne A, Malone PS. The MACE procedure: experience in the United Kingdom. J Pediatr Surg. 1999;34(2):338–40.
4. Van Savage JG, Yohannes P. Laparoscopic antegrade continence enema in situ appendix procedure for refractory constipation and overflow fecal incontinence in children with spina bifida. J Urol. 2000;164(3 Pt 2):1084–7.
5. Yardley IE, Pauniaho S-L, Baillie CT, Turnock RR, Coldicutt P, Lamont GL, et al. After the honeymoon comes divorce: long-term use of the antegrade continence enema procedure. J Pediatr Surg. 2009;44(6):1274–7.
6. Malone, P (2022). 'Episode 13: The development of the Antegrade Continence Enema procedure with Mr. Pat Malone', Circumsession, [Podcast] Dec 2022. Available from: https://podcasters.spotify.com/pod/show/circumsessions/episodes/Episode-13–The-development-of-the-Antegrade-Continence-Enema-procedure-with-Mr–Pat-Malone-e1sp5o8

CHAPTER 40

Cystostomie continente trans-appendiculaire dans le traitement des vessies neurologiques [Trans-Appendicular Continent Cystostomy in the Management of the Neurogenic Bladder]

Paul Mitrofanoff

Chirugie Pediatrique 1980; 21(4):297–305
Citations: $n = 692$

ABSTRACT

'Intermittent catheterisation represents one of the best solutions in case of a neurogenic bladder in children. The authors suggest using the appendix in order to create a passage between the skin and the bladder, the tip of the appendix opening into the bladder at the end of an anti-reflux submucosal tunnel and the other end hemmed to the skin. The bladder neck is usually closed in the course of the same operation. From October, 1976 to January, 1979 16 children underwent such a vesicostomy. In another two cases a trans-urethral cystostomy was carried out. Five cases failed owing to inadequate bladder size and required a cutaneous diversion. The continence of the vesicostomy is total and the comfort obtained was excellent for the other 13 cases. Some complications resulted directly from this technique: cutaneous fistula (1 case) and urethral

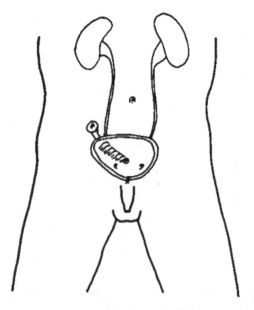

Figure 40.1 Cystostomie continente trans-appendiculaire avec fermeture du col vésical. Disposition finale. (Courtesy of Elsevier Masson.)

DOI: 10.1201/9781003341901-40

repermeation (2 cases). Other problems, common to all conservative treatment of a neurogenic bladder, are discussed: vesico-renal reflux; dilatation of the upper urinary tract; urinary infections; and renal function risk. These appear to be related to a small and hypertonic bladder. These problems must be kept in mind and require strict selection for vesicostomy and careful follow up. (Figure 40.1)'

COMMENTARY (BASHAR ALDEIRI)

Pour notre part, nous avons cherché un procédé qui soit de réalisation suffisamment simple, dont le mécanisme anti-reflux soit efficace et qui soit susceptible de 'tenir' pendant toute une vie

Paul Mitrofanoff started this report by stating, 'We have sought a process which is sufficiently simple to perform, whose antireflux mechanism is effective and which is likely to 'hold' for a lifetime.'

Over four decades have since lapsed, yet the Mitrofanoff concept still holds and still has some time to go.

The technique involved a transverse suprapubic incision to allow extraperitoneal access of the bladder. The peritoneum was widely lifted upwards in order to prepare for an extraperitoneal transposition of the appendix. The peritoneum was then opened in the midline above the bladder, and the appendix was visualised and straightened while preserving the meso-appendix along an appendicular artery pedicle. The appendix was then cut with a caecal cuff, the caecum was closed and the appendix was then extraperitonialised while care was taken not to twist its vascular pedicle. Once this was established, the bladder neck was fully freed as low onto the urethra as possible. The bladder was then opened longitudinally, the ureters were identified and catheterised, and the incision was continued towards the bladder neck. Once at this level, the incision on the bladder neck was made transversely and the urethra and the bladder neck were then closed separately. Further mobilisation of the bladder was then performed to allow it to come as anteriorly as possible towards the abdominal wall. The tip of the appendix was then implanted with an antireflux submucosal tunnel into the right side of the bladder. The ureteral catheters were removed and the bladder was closed all the way down to the old posterior lip of the bladder neck. The bladder was anchored to the posterior rectus sheath, and the appendix was delivered to the skin in a passage through the rectus muscle. A mucocutaneous stoma was then created and a size 10 or 14 F Foley catheter was left in the channel for two weeks.

One of the milestones in achieving social urinary continence was the introduction of clean intermittent catheterisation by Jack Lapides, from Ann Arbor Michigan, in 1972 (1). This concept proved very successful in obtaining continence in cases of overactive bladders and urge incontinence which otherwise maintain a competent bladder neck.

Of course, Mitrofanoff's original paper was published in French and did not gain much notice outside France. It was only when John Duckett of Children's Hospital of Philadelphia embraced and modified the Mitrofanoff concept that the procedure gained any kind of acceptance (2). Duckett's variation of the Mitrofanoff abandoned bladder neck closure and exclusively used the appendix as a conduit.

Mitrofanoff's concept has subsequently led to the introduction of a plethora of alternative conduits to gain access to the bladder, such as the transverse ileal (Yange-Monti) tube, Fallopian tube, tubularised preputial transverse island flaps and longitudinally tubularised ileal and gastric segments.

Intermittent catheterisation was achieved using a 12F, 40 cm long Nelaton catheter. On average, six per day were necessary, and a nocturnal drainage was sometimes carried out. Most children felt an 'urge' before the scheduled catheterisation, which occasionally required a separate catheterisation.

REFERENCES

1. Lapides J, Diokno AC, Silber SJ, Lowe BS. Clean, intermittent self-catheterization in the treatment of urinary tract disease. J Urol. 1972;107:458–461.
2. Duckett JW, Snyder HM 3rd. Continent urinary diversion: variations on the Mitrofanoff principle. J Urol. 1986;136(1):58–62.

CHAPTER 41

The Role of Testicular Vascular Anatomy in the Salvage of High Undescended Testis

Robert Fowler Jr and F Douglas Stephens

Australia and New Zealand Journal of Surgery 1959; 29:92–106
Citations: *n* = 288

ABSTRACT

There are a number of high undescended testes which cannot be brought without tension to the scrotum by conventional techniques of orchidopexy. Most of these testicles suffer an unsatisfactory surgical fate, whether by orchidectomy, abdominal reposition, multiple stage orchidopexy, or ill-advised efforts to secure scrotal fixation under tension. As a group, they present a special problem in management which has received only scant attention in the literature and to which no generally acceptable solution has been found.

The aim of the present investigation has been to refocus attention on high undescended testes and to find a means of reducing the heavy testicular wastage within this group. This paper presents our experience with one method of treatment by which their rate of salvage can be increased. Because the successful application of this method demands a more intimate knowledge of testicular vascular anatomy than is currently available in the surgical literature, this anatomy is presented in some detail. Its importance, moreover, is relevant not only to the mobilization of high undescended testes, but also to an unsuspected by avoidable source of wastage among those testes which can be brought without difficulty to the scrotum.' (Figure 41.1)

COMMENTARY (JOE DAVIDSON)

The Fowler-Stephens approach to intra-abdominal testis represents a true culture shift in the approach of this condition. The two authors, publishing out of the Royal Children's Hospital in Melbourne, Australia, presented what was, at the time, something of a scandalous procedure involving division of the testicular vessels in order to gain sufficient length on the testicular cord to achieve a scrotal position.

They present an expert summary of the literature on testicular vascularisation in the first half of their paper, with particular reverence to the studies of Owen Wangensteen (University of Minnesota Medical School) and Professor RG Harrison (Anatomy Department of the University of Liverpool) (1–3). They also make reference to the early experimental evidence of Dr K Koyano of the University of Kyoto, which had

DOI: 10.1201/9781003341901-41

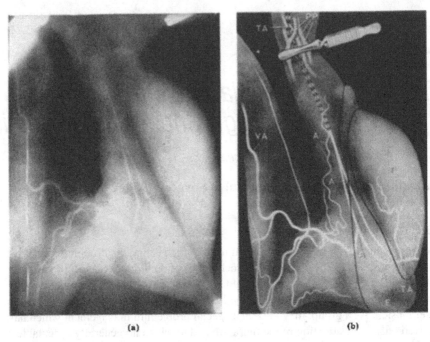

Figure 41.1 M.D., age 11 years and six months. Operative angiogram-retrograde filling from the vassal artery. (a) Photograph of angiogram, and (b) retouched photograph. The testicular artery (T.A. lower) and sundry anastomoses (A) are filled from the vasal artery (V.A.), testis (T.) and epididymis (E.). The clamp is shown compressing the testicular artery (T.A. upper) and the pampiniform plexus of veins (P.P.): the dotted lines represent the unfilled segment of testicular artery above and below the clamp.

been somewhat 'overshadowed in Anglo-Saxon literature'(4). Summarising these anatomic and experimental studies, Fowler and Stephens emphasise the presence of functionally significant arterial anastomoses between the testicular artery and those of the vas deferens and cremaster muscle that are able to provide sufficient blood flow to the testis itself (5). They also draw upon multiple reports from the adult literature whereby radical treatment of recurrent inguinal hernia, mass ligation for varicocele and ligation of the testicular artery in the surgical removal of renal tumours do not appear to result in testicular atrophy in the majority of cases. The authors summarise these observations to reinforce that a ligation should be made as high as possible to avoid disturbing any anastomotic arcades.

The original procedure that was described clearly employed an open, inguinal approach and was performed in a single stage. Since, at the time, there had been no confirmation that an undescended testis possessed the same functional vascular anatomy as had been observed, the authors performed a number of tests intraoperatively – including angiography through the divided inferior epigastric artery and assessment of arterial bleeding from the testis while occluding the testicular artery. The results represent a follow-up ranging from four to 24 months and demonstrated a 'satisfactory' result of a scrotal testis of similar size in eight of 12 cases. Further scrutiny of their case series would reveal that failure was seen in cases where the testis was smallest and already 'flabby' or 'atrophic'. The angiography also provided an important finding of the postanastomotic end vessels, which run superficially beneath the tunica albuginea with variable course and are therefore at risk whenever an 'anchoring' suture might be placed to hold the testicle in the scrotum.

The Fowler-Stephens procedure has evolved over the years in a number of ways. Firstly, a two-stage procedure is now probably the norm (6), as was described initially by Philip Ransley from Great Ormond Street Hospital in London. This appeared to have superior outcomes, with salvage rates approaching 90% in many series (7), although large, single-surgeon series with a one-stage approach series seemed comparable (8). Laparoscopy was clearly an advance diagnostically but has also facilitated high-ligation of the vessels without extensive retroperitoneal dissection. More recently, an alternative technique of anchoring the testis to the opposite anterolateral abdominal wall with vessels intact has been described by Shehata (9). This relies on gradual stretching of the vas and vessels over time, and early adopters of this technique have reported equivalent results (10).

REFERENCES

1. Wangensteen OH. The undescended testis: An experimental and clinical study. Arch Surg. 1927;14:663.
2. Harrison RG, Barclay AE. The distribution of the testicular artery (internal spermatic artery) to the human testis. Br J Urol. 1948;20:57–66.
3. Harrison RG. The comparative anatomy of the blood-supply of the mammalian testis. Proc Zool Soc Lond. 1949;119:325–344.
4. Koyano K. Changes in testes from disturbance in circulation. Aera Sch Med Univ Imp Kioto. 1923;5:275.
5. Harrison RG. The distribution of the vasal and cremasteric arteries to the testis and their functional importance. J Anat. 1949;83:267–282.
6. Ransley PG, Vordermark JS, Caldamone AA, Bellinger MF. Preliminary ligation of the gonadal vessels prior to orchidopexy for the intra-abdominal testicle. World J Urol. 1984;2:266–268.
7. Yu C. Long C, Wei Y, et al. Evaluation of Fowler–Stephens orchiopexy for high-level intra-abdominal cryptorchidism: A systematic review and meta-analysis. Inter J Surg. 2018;60:74–87.
8. Wu CQ, Kirsch AJ. Revisiting the success rate of one-stage Fowler-Stephens orchiopexy with postoperative Doppler ultrasound and long-term follow-up: A 15-year single-surgeon experience. J Pediatr Urol. 2020;16:48–54.
9. Shehata S. Laparoscopically assisted gradual controlled traction on the testicular vessels: a new concept in the management of abdominal testis. A preliminary report. Eur J Pediatr Surg. 2008;18:402–406.
10. Tian Q, Zhou X, Zhang C, et al. Compared outcomes of high-level cryptorchidism managed by Fowler-Stephens orchiopexy versus the Shehata technique: A systematic review and meta-analysis. J Pediatr Urol. 2023. doi:10.1016/j.jpurol.2023.02.025

CHAPTER 42

Metronidazole in Prevention and Treatment of Bacteroides Infections after Appendicectomy

Willis AT, Ferguson IR, Jones PH, Phillips KD, Tearle PV, Berry RB, Fiddian RV, Graham DF, Harland DH, Innes DB, Mee WM, Rothwell-Jackson RL, Sutch I, Kilbey C, and Edwards D

British Medical Journal 1976; 1(6005):318–321.
Citations: $n = 130$

ABSTRACT

This is a strange paper from an unusual part of the world, not usually associated with the medical literature, Luton, a small commuter town to the north of London in the UK. It is included here because appendicitis is such a common event in children, who are subject to the same complications as adults. Yet there are very few therapeutic trials in this population.

This was a double-blind randomized controlled trial in acute appendicitis between 49 patients who received prophylactic metronidazole (1G tds, or 0.5G tds for children, in the form of a rectal suppository) and 46 who received placebo. The full age range was included, even children < 10 years of age.

Anaerobic infection developed in nine (19%) patients in the placebo group with foul-smelling wound discharge and fever, which in five were later treated with metronidazole with resolution. None of the prophylactic group developed anaerobic infection, though five did develop infection (usually superficial) due to *E. coli*, *enterococci* etc. The anaerobic organisms were predominantly *Bacteroides fragilis* and *melaninogenicus*. Retrospective study showed that all those developing infection had peritoneal contamination with anaerobic organisms at the end of surgery and most had gangrenous appendicitis or had technically difficult surgery.

There were no side effects, and administration was 'acceptable to patients'.

COMMENTARY (MARK DAVENPORT)

This is a trial of its time, long before CONSORT guidelines were invented. There were no power calculations, relatively small numbers, no declared or defined primary

 DOI: 10.1201/9781003341901-42

outcomes and in hindsight remarkably nothing other than a placebo was used in the controls. Indeed, the (incomplete) statistical analysis of the numbers is given in the discussion rather than the results section. Up until the 1970s, all sorts of interventions had been suggested as useful to prevent infections in appendicitis. Topical antibiotics (e.g., tetracyclines, noxythioline, polybactrin) and antiseptics (e.g., povidone iodine, chlohexadine) seemed to be in fashion, and ampicillin was usually the intravenous alternative. Some surgeons even encouraged leaving the skin open and unsutured in complicated cases with delay of a few days before definitive closure.

What it did do was emphasise the role of a hitherto ignored part of the bacterial spectrum the anaerobic bacteria. These after all make up about 99% of all bacteria in the gut but historically were hard to culture. *E. coli*, though making up about 0.1% of the gut microbiome, is relatively easy to culture and has been known about for over 100 years. Metronidazole had also been around a long time for the treatment of various parasitical organisms but only relatively recently was identified as effective for this class of bacteria as well as having no effect on aerobic organisms.

More randomized trials (1–3) followed proving the concept, and even in the laparoscopic era metronidazole is still in common use, often in combination with cephalosporins and often as a single daily dose (4). Now, the key concept is, do we actually need an operation in uncomplicated appendicitis? (See Chapter 43.)

REFERENCES

1. Bates T, Touquet VL, Tutton MK, Mahmoud SE, Reuther JW. Prophylactic metronidazole in appendicectomy: a controlled trial. Br J Surg. 1980;67(8):547–50. doi:10.1002/bjs. 1800670805. PMID: 7000227.
2. Busuttil RW, Davidson RK, Fine M, Tompkins RK. Effect of prophylactic antibiotics in acute nonperforated appendicitis: a prospective, randomized, double-blind clinical study. Ann Surg. 1981;194(4):502–09
3. Chiam HL, Chee CP, Cheah KC, Somasundaram K, Puthucheary SD. The prevention of postappendicectomy sepsis by metronidazole and cotrimoxazole: a controlled double blind trial. Aust Nz J Surg. 1983;53(5):421–25.
4. St Peter SD, Tsao K, Spilde TL, Holcomb GW 3rd, Sharp SW, Murphy JP, Snyder CL, Sharp RJ, Andrews WS, Ostlie DJ. Single daily dosing ceftriaxone and metronidazole vs standard triple antibiotic regimen for perforated appendicitis in children: a prospective randomized trial. J Pediatr Surg. 2008;43(6):981–85.

CHAPTER 43

Nonoperative Treatment with Antibiotics versus Surgery for Acute Nonperforated Appendicitis in Children
A Pilot Randomized Controlled Trial

Svensson JF, Patkova B, Almström M, Naji H, Hall NJ, Eaton S, Pierro A, and Wester T

Annals of Surgery 2015; 261(1):67–71.
Citations: $n = 219$

ABSTRACT

Objective: The aim of this study was to evaluate the feasibility and safety of nonoperative treatment of acute nonperforated appendicitis with antibiotics in children.

Methods: A pilot randomized controlled trial was performed comparing nonoperative treatment with antibiotics versus surgery for acute appendicitis in children. Patients with imaging-confirmed acute nonperforated appendicitis who would normally have had emergency appendectomy were randomized either to treatment with antibiotics or to surgery. Follow-up was for one year.

Results: Fifty patients were enrolled; 26 were randomized to surgery and 24 to nonoperative treatment with antibiotics. All children in the surgery group had histopathologically confirmed acute appendicitis, and there were no significant complications in this group. Two of 24 patients in the nonoperative treatment group had appendectomy within the time of primary antibiotic treatment and one patient after nine months for recurrent acute appendicitis. Another six patients have had an appendectomy due to recurrent abdominal pain ($n = 5$) or parental wish ($n = 1$) during the follow-up period; none of these six patients had evidence of appendicitis on histopathological examination.

Conclusions: Twenty-two of 24 patients (92%) treated with antibiotics had initial resolution of symptoms. Of these 22, only one patient (5%) had recurrence of acute appendicitis during follow-up. Overall, 62% of patients have not had an appendectomy during the follow-up period. This pilot trial suggests that nonoperative treatment of acute appendicitis in children is feasible and safe and that further investigation of nonoperative treatment is warranted.

DOI: 10.1201/9781003341901-43

COMMENTARY (JOE DAVIDSON)

Discounting circumcision, trephination and bone setting, appendicectomy is one of the oldest surgical procedures described, with the first deliberate procedure described by Claudius Amyand in London in 1735. It has become one of the most commonly performed abdominal procedures worldwide, and certainly the most commonly performed emergency procedure in both paediatric and adult general surgical practice (1). Famously dismissed by Charles Darwin as a 'useless' organ based on its 'small size and variability in man' (2), the appendix is now recognised to play a role in intestinal immune and microbial homeostasis, so that incidental and prophylactic appendicectomies are generally avoided and there is now an emerging push towards avoiding it as part of the Ladd procedure for malrotation (3, 4).

Given that the appendix appears, indeed, not to be 'useless', the risks of intra-abdominal surgery and that the appendicitis is in fact amenable to nonoperative treatment (5), there has long been a need for high-quality studies to be performed in a paediatric population to identify the treatment efficacy compared to surgical management. Paediatric surgeons must assume practice based on adult data with caution for several reasons. For example, the follow-up duration among our patients is now routinely measured in decades, not years; furthermore, long inpatient stays and illness duration may pose a considerable burden upon caregivers and siblings as well as the patient's own education and social development.

Svensson et al. completed the first randomized controlled trial in children comparing standard surgical management with antibiotic therapy alone. This was a pilot trial, aiming to demonstrate feasibility and safety and produce data upon which a larger study could be designed. At the point of enrolment, all children had undergone imaging in the form of an ultrasound, with CT being performed in cases of diagnostic uncertainty. The primary outcome was defined as 'resolution of symptoms without complication'; surgery was performed with three-port laparoscopy while antibiotic therapy was delivered intravenously for 48 hours minimum and for a total of ten days. Ultimately, almost two thirds (62%) of nonoperative management cases had not undergone an appendicectomy at one year following inclusion; scrutiny of cases who *did* have an appendicectomy in this follow-up period reveals that, in fact, only two were indicated for acute appendicitis. There was one reported case of perforated appendicitis in the nonoperative group, in a child presenting on day nine following initial successful management and discharge.

Debate has raged for some time about the appropriateness of offering nonoperative management for appendicitis at all. Some surgeons argue that appendicectomy is safe, simple and curative, while others argue that the complications from surgery are not insignificant and that a safe option to avoid surgery may be preferable to some, even if it has a relatively high risk of failure. Interestingly, when both patient and surgeon preference are removed from the equation, such as during the COVID-19 pandemic, selective nonoperative management of appendicitis has been shown to be effective with very few negative appendicectomies and low readmission rates across a national cohort reported from the UK (6).

There are still ongoing issues surrounding the correct classification of uncomplicated cases. Various scoring systems based on clinical, biochemical and imaging data have been proposed, but none have been shown to be sufficiently discriminant to merit widespread adoption (7). There are additional benefits of diagnostic imaging, such as reducing unnecessary management (surgical or nonoperative) alongside detection of an associated appendicolith which appears to predict failure of the nonoperative group (8, 9). However, based on this randomized trial and subsequent data that have emerged, nonoperative management of appendicitis ought to feature in the consent process for any child with uncomplicated appendicitis, irrespective of the surgeon's personal preferences and beliefs about its effectiveness.

REFERENCES

1. Scott JW, Olufajo OA, Brat GA, et al. Use of national burden to define operative emergency general surgery. JAMA Surg. 2016;151:e160480.
2. Darwin C. The Descent of Man and Selection in Relation to Sex. 1872.
3. Lukish J, Levitt M, Burd RS, Kane T, Sandler T. More evidence against appendectomy at the time of a Ladd procedure. J Pediatr Surg. 2022;57:751.
4. Davidson JR, Eaton S, De Coppi P. Let sleeping dogs lie: to leave the appendix at the time of a Ladd procedure. J Pediatr Surg. 2017. doi: 10.1016/j.jpedsurg.2017.09.003.
5. de Almeida Leite RM, Seo DJ, Gomez-Eslava B, et al. Nonoperative vs operative management of uncomplicated acute appendicitis: a systematic review and meta-analysis. JAMA Surg. 2022;157(9):828–834.
6. Bethell GS, Gosling T, Rees CM, et al. Impact of the COVID-19 pandemic on management and outcomes of children with appendicitis: the Children with AppendicitiS during the CoronAvirus panDEmic (CASCADE) study. J Pediatr Surg. 2022;57:380–385.
7. RIFT study group et al. Appendicitis risk prediction models in children presenting with right iliac fossa pain (RIFT study): a prospective, multicentre validation study. Lancet Child Adolesc Health. 2020;4:271–280.
8. Tanaka Y, Uchida H, Kawashima H, et al. Long-term outcomes of operative versus nonoperative treatment for uncomplicated appendicitis. J Pediatr Surg. 2015;50:1893–1897.
9. Mahida JB, Lodwick DL, Nacion KM, et al. High failure rate of nonoperative management of acute appendicitis with an appendicolith in children. J Pediatr Surg. 2016;51:908–911.

CHAPTER 44

Long-Term Total Parenteral Nutrition with Growth, Development, and Positive Nitrogen Balance

Stanley J Dudrick, Douglas W Wilmore, Harry M Vars, and Jonathan E Rhoads

Surgery. 1968; 64(1):134–142.
Citations: *n* = 932

ABSTRACT

This paper is an experimental and follow-up clinical study showing that normal life could be sustained using parenteral means only.

The experimental element involved six beagle puppies who were paired after weaning at eight weeks of age with control littermates. Then, at 12 weeks a vinyl catheter was inserted into an external jugular vein and threaded to the superior vena cava. The end was tunnelled to be brought out on the back between the scapulae and the puppies' attached to a harness in a 'metabolic' cage.

These were then fed entirely intravenously for 72–256 days. Their hyperosmolar fluid consisted of high doses of glucose, protein (fibrin) hydrolysate and sometimes fat to provide adequate calories (estimated 140 Kcal/kg/day) and protein (4 gm/kg/day).

The IV puppies actually outstripped their littermates for weight gain and growth (Figure 44.1).

The clinical element described 30 patients with chronic complicated gastrointestinal disease that had been supported exclusively intravenously with 2,400–4,500 Kcals/day for ten to 200 days (Figure 44.2). The most dramatic result of total IV nutrition was the observed normal growth in the children. The best example of this was a 1.8 kg infant with near-total small bowel atresia. During the first 44 days, when there was no possibility of enteral feeding and only total parenteral 'alimentation', the infant gained 1.4 kg of weight and 6.3 cm of length. This patient was also described in an earlier case report published in the *Journal of the American Medical Association* (*JAMA*) in that same year (Wilmore DW, Dudrick SJ. Growth and development of an infant receiving all nutrients exclusively by vein. *JAMA*, 1968, 203:860–864 – cited by 55 papers).

DOI: 10.1201/9781003341901-44

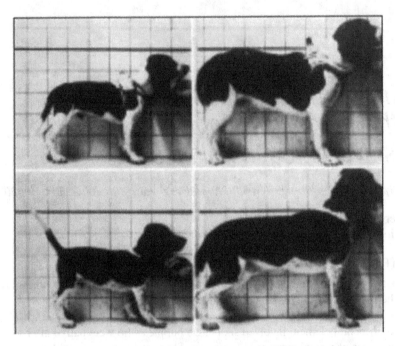

Figure 44.1   Reprinted with permission from Oxford University Press.

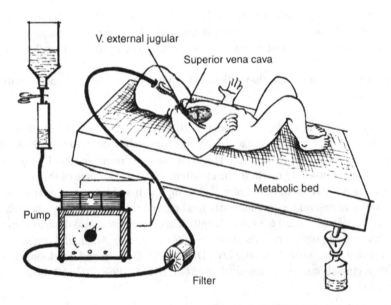

Figure 44.2   Reproduced with permission from JAMA. 1968. Vol. 203 (10): 860–864.

COMMENTARY (MARK DAVENPORT)

Stanley Dudrick was a surgical resident working at the University of Pennsylvania in 1967 with his mentor Jonathan Rhoads (1907–2002). They postulated the not unreasonable notion that to get enough calories in, then you had to concentrate the solution and therefore had to have it infusing in a high-flow central vein to avoid irritant damage to the vein wall. This was a simple concept but a bit more difficult to achieve in real life, so he used fine PVC catheters from the auto industry, firstly in puppies to prove the principle and then later on a series of adults with enteral failure and memorably the baby described in the preceding abstract.

Although glucose and protein were provided, there were no intravenous fat emulsions available at that time, and the infusions were administered by a pump over 24 hours. Following this there was a rapid expansion of the field of parenteral nutrition which coupled with the development of more secure silicone-based intravenous lines increased the survival of many infants with short bowel syndrome.

Stanley Dudrick died recently in 2020, aged 84 years, and never patented any of his inventions, which clearly contributed to the spread of his ideas. He became the first president and founder of the American Society for Parenteral and Enteral Nutrition. Jonathan Rhoads, an adult cancer surgeon, had an equally prestigious career editing the *Annals of Surgery* and writing the *Rhoads' Textbook of Surgery*. Somewhat ironically, towards the end of his life, with the development of stomach cancer and unable to eat, he was maintained for three months on parenteral nutrition.

CHAPTER 45

Splenic Studies. I. Susceptibility to Infection after Splenectomy Performed in Infancy

SPLENIC STUDIES

I. SUSCEPTIBILITY TO INFECTION AFTER SPLENECTOMY PERFORMED IN INFANCY[*]

HAROLD KING, M.D., AND HARRIS B. SHUMACKER, JR., M.D.

INDIANAPOLIS, IND.

FROM THE DEPARTMENT OF SURGERY, INDIANA UNIVERSITY MEDICAL CENTER, INDIANAPOLIS

Annals of Surgery. 1952; 136(2):239–242.
Citations: $n = 774$

ABSTRACT

This paper described the consequences of splenectomy with reference to five infants where it was performed at Indiana Medical Center in the 1950s. Rather like the phenomenon it was describing, it came out as a thunderbolt from a clear blue sky. The authors found only one other possible report in a preterm infant, who had a splenectomy for acute thromocytopaenic purpura in the first few days of life and died from sepsis on the 21st day postoperatively.

In their series, all five infants had had a splenectomy for haemolytic anaemia at varying ages ranging from a few days to five months. They then all had to be readmitted at some future point with varying degrees of sepsis. This included two with proven meningococcal sepsis, from which one died; one with Haemophilus influenza meningitis; one with meningitis? cause; and the final one who died at three months with what proved to be a fatal acute septic event, but no cause was found and a postmortem was not done. In one of the infants who died, infarcted haemorrhagic adrenals were also noted (Waterhouse–Friderchsen syndrome).

Their review highlighted certain experimental studies which emphasised the key role the spleen played in combatting infection, such as Morris and Bullock's study on splenectomised immature rats, where 85% developed fatal sepsis due to Bacterium

DOI: 10.1201/9781003341901-45

enteritidis within two months of surgery. They also relate that if the splenectomy occurred in older children or adults, then no such predisposition was seen.

There was an addendum to the paper that said that no deaths had been seen in a similar series of infancy splenectomies from Boston Children's Hospital, but that it had also been observed in other American hospitals.

COMMENTARY (MARK DAVENPORT)

This paper was followed by several publications particularly from North America arguing vociferously as to whether the King and Schumaker observations were simply bad luck or represented a real risk. This debate and previous reporting were summarised in an article in the *Lancet* in 1962 by Lowden et al. (1) from the northeast of England, reporting their own experiences with 75 children. Severe sepsis developed in four, none over the age of ten years. All were of sudden onset, reaching a rapid crescendo within hours. In three, pneumococcal infection was identified, though only one of them had their spleens removed during infancy; for the other two, this had happened later during childhood. Two of these patients died.

The term 'overwhelming postsplenectomy infection' (OPSI) was later introduced to highlight the dangers of splenectomy, and clinicians moved towards prophylactic measures to limit risk. Current recommendations highlight the role of prophylactic vaccinations specifically directed at the pneumococcus (*Streptococcus pneumoniae*) (e.g., 13-valent pneumococcal conjugate vaccine [PCV13 Prevnar 13™ Pfizer]), the meningococcus (*Neisseria meningitidis*) (e.g., meningococcal ACWY conjugate vaccine [MenACWY™ Sanofi Pasteur] and meningococcal B vaccine [MenB, Bexsero™ Novartis]), and invasive *Haemophilus influenza* (HiB, Menitorix™ GSK). All of these bacteria are encapsulated organisms that thrive due to the lack of protection normally provided by splenic macrophages and the process of opsonisation. Asplenic patients are also more susceptible to other more tropical diseases such as malaria (Falciparum spp.) and babesiosis (*Babesia microti*).

Daily prophylactic oral antibiotics (e.g., penicillin V) are also recommended for all children, potentially forever.

REFERENCE

1. Lowdon AG, Walker JH, Walker W. Infection following splenectomy in childhood. Lancet. 1962;1(7228):499–504.

CHAPTER 46

Sacrococcygeal Teratoma: American Academy of Pediatrics Surgical Section Survey-1973

R Peter Altman, Judson G Randolph, and John R Lilly

Journal of Pediatric Surgery 1974; 9(3):389–398.
Citations: *n* = 594

ABSTRACT

'This report was compiled from a survey of the membership of the Surgical Section of the American Academy of Pediatrics. Details pertinent to the experience with sacrococcygeal teratoma for the ten-year period 1962–1972 were requested in a questionnaire circulated to the full membership. The data from 405 clinical cases have been tabulated and constitute the basis of this report. Included among the 81 responses received were institutional reports reviewing the experience of several surgeons as well as case material submitted by individuals.'

COMMENTARY (MARK DAVENPORT)

Sacrococcygeal tumours (SCT) are the commonest of the tumours that present at birth, and many are all too obvious presenting a challenging surgical problem with perhaps an uncertain outcome. This report by the Surgical Section of the oldest American paediatric surgical society defined the disease in the days before the availability of antenatal ultrasound. It is actually a mammoth undertaking involving a survey of all the members (but how many and from where is not really made clear) but is without any confirmation of accuracy or reliability of data. There is a reference to the use of a computer in managing the data – probably a first.

The study is based upon 405 (mostly female) cases, of which 225 presented as neonates. The classification is the study's best remembered legacy and divides them into Type I (*n* = 186, 46%), II (*n* = 138, 34%), III (*n* = 35, 8.6%) and IV (*n* = 39, 9.6%) (illustrated in Figure 46.1). They recognised that evidence of malignancy (distant metastases, *n* = 18) bore a strong relationship with both the type of SCT (Type 1–0%, Type 2–6%, Type 3–20% and Type 4–8%) and time of presentation (average age 22 months).

Surgery was typically single-stage from below (314/395, 79.5%), but 52 (13.1%) required an additional abdominal approach (one- or two-stage).

   DOI: 10.1201/9781003341901-46

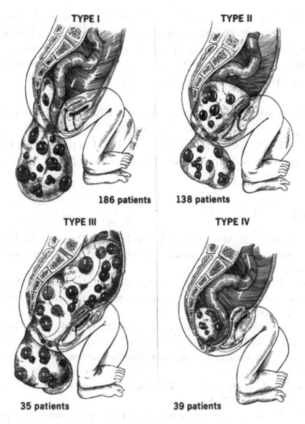

Figure 46.1 Classification of Sacro-coccygeal teratomas.

Mortality was significant, ranging from 11% of Type I tumours to 28% of Type III tumours. Although deaths were common with those defined as malignant, it was also seen in the large (> 10 cms) tumours even if histologically benign. Actual morbidity was not really described here, though urinary diversion and colostomy was required in 3.2% and 4.7% respectively.

The importance of a coccygectomy in reducing recurrence rates became part of surgical dogma after this paper, though where it originated from is not clear. Since that era, much of the focus has changed to that of the antenatal period, probably starting in the 1980s. Nowadays this is where much of the mortality is observed, and this would not have been evident to surgeons in the 1960s and 1970s. One study, published in 2006, from a large fetal medicine centre with 100% antenatal detection quotes an overall survival of 77% (1). Antenatal intervention is now possible from tumour debulking at open fetal surgery (2) to less invasive interventions such as recurrent cyst aspiration and parenchymal debulking using *in utero* lasers or alcohol injection (3). Surgical resection of the larger ones is still challenging, and although deaths are rare, morbidity can still be seen, although how much is still debated.

A series from Great Ormond Street, London, from the 1970s and 1980s (4) suggested that up to 40% of survivors had incontinence (urine and faecal) or locomotor issues and was mirrored by a Dutch National study (5) in 2007 and even in a long-term study from Philadelphia, Pennsylvania, in 2014 (6). However, nothing like this was seen in the King's College Hospital series referred to earlier (1).

All three authors of this landmark paper worked at Children's Hospital Medical Center, Washington, DC, with Judson Randolph (1927–2015) being the chief and Peter Altman (1934– 2011) and John Lilly (1929–1995) as the juniors. Both of these later headed influential paediatric surgical departments in New York and Denver respectively.

REFERENCES

1. Makin EC, Hyett J, Ade-Ajayi N, Patel S, Nicolaides K, Davenport M. Outcome of antenatally diagnosed sacrococcygeal teratomas: single-center experience (1993-2004). J Pediatr Surg. 2006;41(2):388–93.
2. Hedrick HL, Flake AW, Crombleholme TM, Howell LJ, Johnson MP, Wilson RD, Adzick NS. Sacrococcygeal teratoma: prenatal assessment, fetal intervention, and outcome. J Pediatr Surg. 2004;39(3):430–38.
3. Sananes N, Javadian P, Schwach Werneck Britto I, Meyer N, Koch A, Gaudineau A, Favre R, Ruano R. Technical aspects and effectiveness of percutaneous fetal therapies for large sacrococcygeal teratomas: cohort study and literature review. Ultrasound Obstet Gynecol. 2016;47(6):712–19.
4. Malone PS, Spitz L, Kiely EM, et al. The functional sequelae of sacrococcygeal teratoma. J Pediatr Surg. 1990;25:679–80.
5. Derikx JP, De Backer A, van de Schoot L, et al. Long-term functional sequelae of sacrococcygeal teratoma: a national study in the Netherlands. J Pediatr Surg. 2007;42(6):1122–26.
6. Partridge EA, Canning D, Long C, et al. Urologic and anorectal complications of sacrococcygeal teratomas: prenatal and postnatal predictors. J Pediatr Surg. 2014;49(1):139–42.

CHAPTER 47

Mortality from Gastrointestinal Congenital Anomalies at 264 Hospitals in 74 Low-Income, Middle-Income, and High-Income Countries A Multicentre, International, Prospective Cohort Study

Global PaedSurg Research Collaboration (Naomi J Wright, Andrew JM Leather, Niyi Ade-Ajayi, et al.)

Lancet. 2021 July 24; 398(10297):325–339.
Citations: *n* = 29

ABSTRACT

This is a multicentre, international prospective cohort study of 3,849 patients (< 16 years), presenting to 264 hospitals in 74 countries around the world (high-income [*n* = 89]; middle-income [*n* = 166] and low-income countries [*n* = 9]) between October 2018 and April 2019. The main conditions were congenital gastrointestinal in origin and included oesophageal atresia (*n* = 560); congenital diaphragmatic hernia (*n* = 448); intestinal atresia (*n* = 681); gastroschisis (*n* = 453); exomphalos (*n* = 325); anorectal malformation (*n* = 991); and Hirschsprung's disease (*n* = 517).

There were obvious differences in mortality, e.g., all conditions 37 (39·8%) of 93 in low-income countries (LIC), 583 (20·4%) of 2,860 in middle-income countries (MIC) and 50 (5·6%) of 896 in high-income countries (HIC) (p < 0·0001), with gastroschisis being the most disparate (Figure 47.1). Poor prognostic factors included sepsis at presentation and the unavailability of ventilation, parenteral nutrition and peripherally inserted central venous catheters when needed.

Antenatal diagnosis was rare in LIC (9/93 (9·7%) versus 823/2860 (28·8%) (MIC) versus 506/896 (56·5%) (HIC), and most were born via vaginal delivery (80·7% vs 49·7% vs 45·8%).

DOI: 10.1201/9781003341901-47

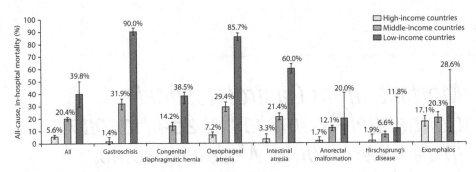

Figure 47.1 Difference in mortality for typical neonatal surgical conditions according to national economic status. (Courtesy of the Lancet, open access.)

This study aimed to form a realistic baseline and framework for a renewed push towards improving 'unacceptable' mortality simply due to global inequality.

COMMENTARY (NAOMI WRIGHT)

Neonates now comprise 46% of the 5.2 million annual global deaths in children under five years of age. Congenital anomalies have risen to become the fifth leading cause of death in children under five years, with over 95% of the half a million annual deaths from these conditions occurring in low- and middle-income countries (LMICs). Gastrointestinal congenital anomalies likely contribute to a significant proportion of this mortality, as they are commonly lethal without access to emergency neonatal surgical care soon after birth. However, very little was known about the outcomes of these conditions in LMICs. Hence, we decided to undertake the Global PaedSurg study, the first international prospective cohort study comparing outcomes from seven of the commonest gastrointestinal anomalies in low-, middle- and high-income countries globally.

This idea was born following a PaedSurg Africa study which highlighted a 76% mortality from gastroschisis across sub-Saharan Africa (SSA). It was through the PaedSurg Africa study that we developed the study methodology (inspired by research from the GlobalSurg study group) and the SSA research network. We also used connections from across the world that we had become connected to through the Global Initiative for Children's Surgery (GICS). I started by developing the research protocol with my core PhD supervision team and a select group of experts from across the globe. I then recruited a 'Lead Organising Committee' formed of approximately 30 medical students, juniors doctors and surgeons from PaedSurg Africa, GICS, personal contacts and King's College London (our base). This team was key to managing the logistics of communicating with hundreds of research collaborators from countries across the world. We used six Gmail email accounts specifically set up for the study (with translation facilities), shared online databases and held weekly organising committee meetings via video conference.

I recruited the research collaborators, who contributed the data to the study, through the aforementioned networks, presentations at conferences globally, a study website publicised through social media and through a network of nominated 'Country and Regional Leads' who reached out to children's surgical teams within their respective regions. Collaborators created local research teams, gained institutional ethical approval, took patient consent where required, collected deidentified data and entered it into REDCap and contributed to the subsequent data interpretation and write-up through online video meetings and email communication. To optimise accessibility, we provided all study documentation, email communication, the website and REDCap data collection forms in 12 languages. There was no monetary payment for participation; motivation was provided through a desire to be part of the world's first truly global research study in paediatric surgery and authorship on the resultant publication. We also ran a Research Training Fellowship and Mentorship Scheme, free of charge, for all research collaborators to support them to undertake their own research alongside the main study. Collaborators were key to dissemination of the study results globally through local, national and international presentations; TV reports; newspaper articles; meetings with ministers of health; and development of training modules. It was a truly collaborative international effort.

CHAPTER 48

Tumour Angiogenesis Therapeutic Implications

Judah Folkman

New England Journal of Medicine 1971; 285:1182–1186
Citations: n = 2,928!

ABSTRACT

'The growth of solid neoplasms is always accompanied by neovascularization. This new capillary growth is even more vigorous and continuous than a similar outgrowth of capillary sprouts observed in fresh wounds or in inflammation. Many workers have described the association between growing solid malignant tumours and new vessel growth. However, it has not been appreciated until the past few years that the population of tumour cells and the population of capillary endothelial cells within a neoplasm may constitute a highly integrated ecosystem. In this ecosystem the mitotic index of the two cell populations may depend upon each other. Tumour cells appear to stimulate endothelial-cell proliferation, and endothelial cells may have an indirect effect over the rate of tumour growth.'

COMMENTARY (PAOLO DE COPPI)

Dr Judah Folkman (1933–2008), the father of angiogenesis research, was the director of the Vascular Biology Program and a former surgeon-in-chief at the Children's Hospital Boston. Dr Folkman was certainly one of the most innovative surgeon scientists. Not only had he the ability to innovate the field of paediatric surgery by capturing the most significant problems in our field (i.e., how tumours grow), but he was also unique in answering some of the questions by leading a basic science lab, something almost unheard at the time of his clinical practice. That unique ability to bring together both a scientist's and a surgeon's perspectives to finding solutions has remained unfortunately very rare in our field. Dr Folkman published his ideas about angiogenesis in 1971 in the highlighted landmark paper and showed that tumour expansion required a family of angiogenic regulatory molecules. In the early 1970s, he had preliminary evidence that any proliferating tissue could not enlarge beyond a few millimetres without recruiting new vessels, a concept which has subsequently been validated in many studies and adopted as dogma in regenerative medicine. Interestingly, to support his theories, his laboratory introduced novel techniques and assays which are still valid and performed in regenerative medicine, such cloning capillary endothelial cells in vitro (1) and studying blood vessel outgrowth on the *ex vivo* chicken embryo chorioallantoic membrane (2). In the mid-1990s, Folkman and

DOI: 10.1201/9781003341901-48

colleagues had published a series of papers demonstrating that vascular endothelial growth factor (VEGF) is a critical mediator of retinal neovascularisation, so it would therefore be an appropriate target for antiangiogenic therapy of age-related neovascular macular degeneration (3). In December 2005, *Nature* published a major review of the field of angiogenesis research and predicted that 'angiogenesis research will probably change the face of medicine in the next decades', with more than 500 million people worldwide predicted to benefit from pro- or antiangiogenesis treatments (4).

I was fortune enough to interact with Dr Folkman while a research fellow at Children's Hospital and appreciated the multiple factors that helped such innovative work emerge in Dr Folkman's laboratory. First, he was a very inquisitive man and never stopped pushing his own imagination or the bounds of scientific understanding which permeated all the research fellows and surgeons who worked with him. He used to say, 'Science goes where you imagine it.' He was warm, humble, passionate about teaching and had an unlimited creativity tempered by a vast clinical experience. I was amongst the fortunate who was influenced both directly and indirectly by him and still remember when I first met him in the early 2000s. Despite not being my primary supervisor, he would stop me in the corridor, being genuinely interested in asking about the amniotic stem cells which we were trying to characterise at that time (5). Second, he strongly believed in interactions between different scientific disciplines. Mixing engineers, biologists and surgeons in the same laboratory was certainly a very innovative approach at that time, whereas 'team science' is now a standard that is considered to be absolutely necessary, not only for regenerative medicine but in all translational sciences. Third, while Dr. Folkman was fascinated by angio- and vasculogenesis or the growth of blood vessels occurring during tumour growth, he mentored various scientists and clinicians in his lab that took this idea forward and explored the role of vascular network growth to engineer new tissues. Working together in his laboratory at that time were Dr Jay Vacanti and Dr Robert Langer, who started collaborating to create new matrices and scaffolds that could allow cells to be expanded and to differentiate. They defined the concept of tissue engineering as a new field that applies the principles of biology and engineering to the development of functional substitutes for damaged tissue. Dr Folkman's mentorship influenced many working in Boston at that time, and just a few floors below in the same building Dr Anthony Atala engineered the first human bladder, which was later implanted in children requiring bladder augmentation. As a cascade, generations to follow were fortunate to be trained directly by him and his fellows working in the field of regenerative medicine.

REFERENCES

1. J Folkman, Haudenschild CC, Zetter BR, Long-term culture of capillary endothelial cells. Proc Natl Acad Sci USA. 1979;76:5217–5221.
2. Ausprunk DH, Knighton DR, Folkman J. Differentiation of vascular endothelium in the chick chorioallantois: a structural and autoradiographic study. Dev Biol. 1974;38:237–248.

3. Rosenfeld PJ, Brown DM, Heier JS, et al. Ranibizumab for neovascular age-related macular degeneration. N Engl J Med. 2006;355:1419–1431.
4. Carmeliet P. Angiogenesis in life, disease and medicine. Nature. 2005;438:932–936.
5. De Coppi P, Bartsch G Jr, Siddiqui MM, et al. Isolation of amniotic stem cell lines with potential for therapy. Nat Biotechnol. 2007;25(1):100–106.

EDITOR'S COMMENTARY (JOE DAVIDSON)

In this seminal work, Dr Judah Folkman (1933–2008) begins by introducing the new concept that tumour cells appeared to be able to rapidly induce growth in neighbouring blood vessels and showed elegantly, by wrapping the tumour in a membrane, that this was due to a secreted factor by the cells and not by cell contact. He goes on to discuss the evidence that this isn't an advantageous property of tumour cells but a necessary one; without nearby endothelial cells, tumours will not grow beyond a size of 2–3 mm. Furthermore, the fact that tumour cells tend to outgrow their capillary network further appears to be a major limiting factor to overall tumour growth. Having presented his own and others' observations initially in the paper, Folkman moves on to describe his own experimental findings of a soluble factor that appears to be responsible for endothelial growth, and that the key involvement of the angiogenesis process in early tumour formation and tumour growth might be a key avenue to treat cancer in the future.

Folkman's theory, published in this paper, set the scene for decades of work from his own group and others. He went on to publish many times in the headline journals of biomedical science: *Nature* (1–3), *Science* (4, 5) and *Cell* (6, 7). What was initially dubbed tumour-derived angiogenic factor (TAF) gave way to a family of molecules that are now individually the subject of research for entire groups: vascular endothelial growth factor (VEGF) signalling has been shown to be a crucial component of many conditions from retinopathy of prematurity to neurodegenerative diseases of aging (8). Furthermore, millions of patients worldwide will have received medications aimed at disrupting the angiogenesis pathway. Folkman's observations of the upregulation of angiogenesis pathway in nonsolid tumours led to the approval of thalidomide to be used in patients with multiple myeloma in 1999 (9). A few years later in 2004, the first of several monoclonal antibodies targeting the VEGF pathway emerged with Bevacizumab (Avastin™) receiving FDA approval for use as a first-line treatment of colorectal cancer in 2004, and subsequent approvals were granted for use in many other cancer chemotherapy regimens, specifically demonstrating survival benefits in advanced and metastatic disease (10).

For more than 40 years, Judah Folkman worked tirelessly, exploring tumour vascular biology, creating an entirely new field of science and earning himself the title 'The Father of Angiogenesis'. These were great achievements certainly but not enough apparently to satisfy the requirements of a Nobel Prize committee, which many people thought he deserved.

REFERENCES

1. Ingber D, Fujita T, Kishimoto S, et al. Synthetic analogues of fumagillin that inhibit angiogenesis and suppress tumour growth. Nature. 1990;348:555–557.
2. Holmgren L, O'Reilly MS, Folkman J. Dormancy of micrometastases: balanced proliferation and apoptosis in the presence of angiogenesis suppression. Nature Med. 1995;1:149–153.
3. Folkman J, Watson K, Ingber D, Hanahan D. Induction of angiogenesis during the transition from hyperplasia to neoplasia. Nature. 1989;339:58–61.
4. Folkman J, Langer R, Linhardt RJ, Haudenschild C, Taylor S. Angiogenesis inhibition and tumor regression caused by heparin or a heparin fragment in the presence of cortisone. Science. 1983;221(4612):719–725.
5. O'Reilly MS, Pirie-Shepherd S, Lane WS, Folkman J. Antiangiogenic activity of the cleaved conformation of the serpin antithrombin. Science. 1999;285:1926–1928.
6. O'Reilly MS, Holmgren L, Shing Y, et al. Angiostatin: a novel angiogenesis inhibitor that mediates the suppression of metastases by a Lewis lung carcinoma. Cell. 1994;79:315–328.
7. O'Reilly MS, Boehm T, Shing Y, et al. Endostatin: an endogenous inhibitor of angiogenesis and tumor growth. Cell. 1997;88:277–285.
8. Ferrara N, Henzel WJ. Pituitary follicular cells secrete a novel heparin-binding growth factor specific for vascular endothelial cells. Biochem Biophys Res Commun. 1989;161:851–858.
9. Singhal S, Mehta J, Desikan R, et al. Antitumor activity of thalidomide in refractory multiple myeloma. N Engl J Med. 1999;341:1565–1571.
10. Garcia J, Hurwitz HI, Sandler AB, et al. Bevacizumab (Avastin®) in cancer treatment: a review of 15 years of clinical experience and future outlook. Cancer Treat Rev. 2020;86:102017.

CHAPTER 49

Prolonged Duration of Response to Infliximab in Early but Not Late Paediatric Crohn's Disease

Kugathasan S, Werlin SL, Martinez A, Rivera MT, Heikenen JB, and Binion DG

Am J Gastroenterol. 2000 November;95(11):3189–3194.
Citations: $n = 230$

ABSTRACT

Introduction: Tumour necrosis factor (TNF) alpha plays a central role in chronic intestinal inflammation of Crohn's disease. Targeting this cytokine with the chimeric monoclonal antibody infliximab has emerged as an effective form of therapy in adult Crohn's disease (CD) patients.

Methods: Fifteen consecutive children (mean age 12.8 ± 3.2 years) with medically refractory Crohn's disease were enrolled in a prospective, open-label trial of a single, 5 mg/kg infliximab intravenous infusion. 'Medically refractory disease' was defined as an inability to taper steroids, lack of response to immunomodulator therapy over four months and active disease as measured by the Pediatric Crohn's Disease Activity Index (PCDAI). Primary endpoints included measurements of disease activity (PCDAI), steroid use and duration of clinical response.

Results: In all, 14/15 children (94%) improved after infliximab infusion, with a significant decrease of both PCDAI and daily steroid use by four weeks. Ten patients (67%) achieved complete remission by 10 weeks. Among the 14 patients who responded, three of six children (50%) with early disease maintained clinical response through the 12-month trial period, compared to none of eight children with late disease. There were no serious complications associated with the use of infliximab in any of the patients.

It is important to note that 11/14 of these responders had a clinical relapse within the subsequent year requiring escalation of medical care or surgery – this included all of the patients with late CD, while 50% of the early CD patients were maintained event free on maintenance therapy.

DOI: 10.1201/9781003341901-49

EDITOR'S COMMENTARY (JOE DAVIDSON)

The earliest reports of the use of the anti-TNF monoclonal antibody, cA2, appeared in the mid-1990s (1) and this paper from Milwaukee, Wisconsin, and one from a group in Connecticut (2) first reported the use of Infliximab in children with CD.

Monoclonal antibody therapy against various components of the inflammatory cascade, an entirely new category of drugs, started to emerge during the mid-1980s. Initially, Murmonab-CD3 (aka OKT3) (Orthoclone™) was introduced as an anti-CD3 agent to prevent acute allograft rejection in kidney transplantation. As a partial agonist of the T-cell receptor, infusion of OKT3 led to considerable side effects relating to cytokine release syndrome, and has since been discontinued in preference of other agents with milder side effect profiles. However, this pioneering treatment has led to a wave of monoclonal therapies, with the 100th monoclonal antibody product receiving FDA approval in 2021 (3). Initially these were made from immunised mouse spleen cells that were subsequently fused with cancer cells *in vitro* to give an immortal cell line that would produce the antibody of choice. Other methods of immortalising cells such as viral transfection have since been employed, and chimeric antibodies as well as those from human-derived cells are also readily available. The nomenclature of these products is logical, albeit convoluted, and has recently been reformatted by the World Health Organisation (4).

Since this initial report, there have been several high-quality studies that have followed. The most recent such study was the open-label randomized control trial of first-line infliximab for new-onset CD, published by Jongsma in 2022 (5). The findings of this latest study confirm, with high-quality evidence, the observed benefits of Infliximab in treating new onset disease – with a higher proportion of patients achieving clinical and endoscopic remission compared to conventional therapy and fewer patients needing escalation of their medical management over the year following enrolment.

Looking ahead, Crohn's disease should benefit from advanced understanding of genetic and epigenetic influences as well as advances in understanding of the immune system and metabolome. Cell-adhesion and intracellular signalling pathways are targets for a host of new monoclonal agents (6). The challenge for the future will be recognising the individual nuances of each individual case in order to select truly personalised therapy.

REFERENCES

1. van Dullemen HM, van Deventer SJ, Hommes DW, et al. Treatment of Crohn's disease with anti-tumor necrosis factor chimeric monoclonal antibody (cA2). Gastroenterology. 1995;109(1):129–135.
2. Hyams JS, Markowitz J, Wyllie R. Use of infliximab in the treatment of Crohn's disease in children and adolescents. J Pediatr. 2000;137(2):192–196.

3. Mullard A. FDA approves 100th monoclonal antibody product. Nat Rev Drug Discov. 2021;20:491–495.

4. Balocco R, De Sousa Guimaraes Koch S, Thorpe R, Weisser K, Malan S. New INN nomenclature for monoclonal antibodies. Lancet. 2022;399:24.

5. Jongsma MME, Aardoom MA, Cozijnsen MA, et al. First-line treatment with infliximab versus conventional treatment in children with newly diagnosed moderate-to-severe Crohn's disease: an open-label multicentre randomised controlled trial. Gut. 2022;71:34.

6. Kobayashi T, Hibi T. Improving IBD outcomes in the era of many treatment options. Nat Rev Gastroenterol Hepatol. 2023;20:79–80.

CHAPTER 50

Bowel Function and Gastrointestinal Quality of Life among Adults Operated for Hirschsprung Disease during Childhood: A Population-Based Study

Kristiina Jarvi, Elina M Laitakari, Antti Koivusalo, Risto J Rintala, and Mikko P Pakarinen

Ann Surg 2010 December;252(6):977–981.
Citations: n = 115

ABSTRACT

Background: Outcomes of Hirschsprung disease (HD) extending to adulthood are unclear; bowel function and quality of life may deteriorate during the aging process.

Methods: Bowel function and gastrointestinal quality of life were cross-sectionally assessed in a population-based manner among adults operated for HD during childhood between 1950 and 1986. Patients were interviewed during their outpatient visit. Controls matched for age and sex were randomly chosen from the Population Register Centre of Finland.

Results: Ninety-two (64%) patients representative for the entire study population responded. The mean age of patients (79% male) was 43 (interquartile range [IQR], 35–48) years. Most (78%) had undergone Duhamel operation, and 94% had aganglionosis confined to the rectosigmoid. The mean overall bowel function score was decreased among patients (17.1 ± 2.8 vs 19.1 ± 1.2; $P < 0.0001$). They reported increased incidence of inability to hold back defecation (40% vs 17%), fecal soiling (48% vs 22%), constipation (30% vs 9%) and social problems related to bowel function (29% vs 11%; $P < 0.05$ for all). Gastrointestinal quality of life was only marginally lower among patients (121 ± 15.3 vs 125 ± 13.1; $P = 0.058$) mainly because of significantly lower scores in questions assessing disease-specific factors such as bowel function and continence. Age was the only predictor of poor bowel function (OR 1.07, 95% CI 1.00–1.14, $P = 0.049$), which weakly predicted gastrointestinal quality of life (OR 0.81, 95% CI 0.66–1.01, $P = 0.05$).

Conclusions: Although bowel function deteriorates with increasing age after operated HD, it is associated with only slightly decreased gastrointestinal quality of life.

DOI: 10.1201/9781003341901-50

COMMENTARY (MIKKO PAKARRINEN)

Long-term outcome may be viewed as one of the most relevant quality indicators and the ultimate measure of success of paediatric surgical care. As survival in most paediatric surgical conditions has risen well above 90%, the focus of interest is turning not only towards long-term organ function but also general health and quality of life. Initially successful surgery does not necessarily guarantee the following 80 years will be carefree, which we should actively pursue with the current life expectancy in the Western world. In some paediatric surgical conditions, postoperative functional impairments and underlying genetic etiology may give raise to previously unrecognized long-term complications which manifest only later in life during adulthood. Thus, long-term follow-up studies not only provide ultimate results of surgical treatment but also complete the natural postoperative history of paediatric surgical conditions guiding their management after transition of care to adult medicine.

This was one of the first papers to comprehensively address true long-term outcomes of Hirschsprung's disease in a controlled manner. It was published by Kriistina Kyrklund (under her maiden name of Järvi at the time) and her colleagues from Helsinki. In this study, 92 adults (64% of the total patient population) with mean age of 43 years, who had been operated on for Hirschsprung's disease in childhood, were compared to normal population controls matched for age and sex. Although patients scored worse in overall bowel function and items addressing urgency, fecal soiling and constipation, the proportion of patients with frequent functional problems remained relatively low at around 10%. However, social issues related bowel dysfunction were more frequent, and quality of life assessment revealed harm to sexual life and loss of physical strength in addition to expected quality of life issues related to bowel dysfunction, despite excluding the three patients with colostomy formation in adulthood. These findings highlighted the importance of wider engagement of outcome measures to achieve a realistic view of the bigger picture.

Linkage of accurate and multifaceted healthcare registries as well as personal identification codes for all citizens enable accurate identification and tracking of patients and matched normal population controls for long-term follow-up studies in countries like Finland. Reliability is further increased by equal access to national taxation-funded healthcare. In addition to the preceding study, these premises together with people's generally positive attitude towards healthcare research have provided population-based follow-up of adults with operated oesophageal atresia, unveiling high incidence of epithelial dysplasia underpinned by oesophageal dysmotility (1), as well as characterization of age-specific development of bowel and bladder control in the normal background population for control purposes (2, 3). While performance of long-term follow-up studies with reliable identification of patients and randomly selected matched normal population controls may be more feasible in some countries and healthcare systems than others, inclusion of core long-term outcome sets, including quality of life assessment as part of routine patient follow-up, would greatly increase our understanding of far-reaching consequences of paediatric surgery.

COMMENTARY (JOE DAVIDSON)

Paediatric surgery is rather uniquely poised among other specialities as the only surgical speciality with truly 'lifelong outcomes'. Many congenital conditions we treat were associated with high mortality until advances in neonatal care allowed for laparotomy and thoracotomy to be performed with generally positive outcomes. While specialities such as adult oncologic or cardiac surgery might report long-term outcomes in years, we should be striving to report our outcomes in decades. When considering these studies, certain aspects enable such studies to be performed, including robust and accurate medical records and population registers – unsurprisingly, therefore, it has been the paediatric surgeons of the Nordic region who have really set a standard in long-term outcomes research, none more so than Risto Rintala and Mikko Pakarinen and their team from Helsinki, who have now published outcome data for adult cohorts with a variety of conditions (4–6). What sets this paper apart is that it uses objective outcome measures in the form of the Gastrointestinal Quality of Life Index (GIQLI) (7) and Bowel Function Score (BFS) (8) in a large cohort of patients with HD with healthy controls provided from the general population.

The results they describe reinforce important messages regarding the long-term trajectory of patients with HD after discharge from paediatric services. Although many patients will fall within the 'normal' range for bowel function and quality of life metrics, there are appreciable differences from the normal population. These have been described in later studies from other centres using the same instruments (9, 10). The correlation of functional outcomes and quality of life indicators is an important association to recognise for all surgeons who treat children with lifelong conditions such as HSCR, and appears to be consistent across cohorts with little impact of the surgical approach taken (11). This reinforces the need to engage optimally with adolescent patients and adopt a holistic approach to the process of transition out of paediatric services.

Some decades after Dr H. William Clatworthy wrote (in a letter to his colleague Judson Randolph) on the concept of 'saving lifetimes', surely now we must now study the content and quality of those lifetimes saved, so that we can continue to improve the outcomes of the service we deliver.

REFERENCES

1. Sistonen SJ, Koivusalo A, Nieminen U, et al. Esophageal morbidity and function among adults with repaired esophageal atresia with tracheoesophageal fistula: a population-based long-term follow-up. Ann Surg. 2010;251:1167–73.
2. Kyrklund K, Koivusalo A, Rintala RJ, Pakarinen MP. Evaluation of bowel function and fecal continence in 594 healthy Finnish individuals aged 4-26 years. Dis Colon Rectum. 2012;55:671–76.
3. Kyrklund K, Taskinen S, Rintala RJ, Pakarinen MP. Evaluation of voiding habits and bladder control in 594 healthy Finnish individuals aged 4-26 years. J Urology. 2012;188:588–93.

4. Koivusalo A, Pakarinen M, Vanamo K, Lindahl H, Rintala RJ. Health-related quality of life in adults after repair of congenital diaphragmatic defects–a questionnaire study. J Pediatr Surg. 2005;40:1376–81.

5. Hukkinen M, Ruuska S, Pihlajoki M, et al. Long-term outcomes of biliary atresia patients surviving with their native livers. Best Pract Res Clin Gastroenterol. 2022;56–57:101764.

6. Kyrklund K, Pakarinen MP, Koivusalo A, Rintala RJ. Bowel functional outcomes in females with perineal or vestibular fistula treated with anterior sagittal anorectoplasty. Dis Colon Rectum. 2015;58:97–103.

7. Eypasch E, Williams JI, Wood-Dauphinee S, et al. Gastrointestinal quality of life index: development, validation and application of a new instrument. Br J Surg. 1995;82:216–22.

8. Rintala RJ, Lindahl H. Is normal bowel function possible after repair of intermediate and high anorectal malformations? J Pediatr Surg. 1995;30:491–94.

9. Granström AL, Danielson J, Husberg B, Nordenskjöld A, Wester T. Adult outcomes after surgery for Hirschsprung's disease: evaluation of bowel function and quality of life. J Pediatr Surg. 2015;50:1865–69.

10. Davidson JR, Kyrklund K, Eaton S, et al. Long-term surgical and patient-reported outcomes of Hirschsprung disease. J Pediatr Surg. 2021;56:1502–11.

11. Davidson JR, Mutanen A, Salli M, et al. Comparative cohort study of Duhamel and endorectal pull-through for Hirschsprung's disease. BJS Open. 2022;6(1):zrab143. doi: 10.1093/bjsopen/zrab143

Index

Note: Locators in *italics* represent figures and **bold** indicate tables in the text.

Printed in the United States
by Baker & Taylor Publisher Services

Printed in the United States
by Baker & Taylor Publisher Services